I0413921

# Kitchen Confidence
## Save Money, Improve your Health, Waste Less

A guidebook by Amanda Terillo, RD, MS

To my Dad who listens to my nutrition advice

# Chapter 1: Introduction

## About This Book

Throughout my career as a registered dietitian, I have worked in a variety of community and clinical settings. I have worked with patients of varying ages, education levels, and cultural backgrounds. Many of these patients had diet-related diseases such as heart disease, kidney disease, diabetes, and cancer. They all wanted to eat better, but many of my patients lacked cooking skills, could not find the time to cook or prep, or felt overwhelmed by all the nutrition advice they were receiving. Educating my patients about simple ways to improve their diet was so rewarding. It improved not only their eating habits, but helped their family's eating habits as well.

In addition to being a registered dietitian, I am also an advocate for a sustainable change in our food system, particularly decreasing food waste. I have completed my Master's Degree in Sustainable Food Systems from Green Mountain College. My studies have shown me that food is more than a source of calories. Farming and agriculture play a vital role in our communities and contribute to our health and the environment.

This guidebook gives me the opportunity to combine my knowledge of nutrition with my passion for changing our food system. Eating healthy food, cooking more at home, and being more resourceful in the kitchen will improve your health, save money, and at the same time cut back on food waste.

## What It Will Teach You

This guidebook will teach you how to create a healthy kitchen environment that will ultimately improve your eating habits. In order to make a lifelong sustainable change in your eating habits, you need to focus on the big picture, which is your health. When you become comfortable and confident in the kitchen you will want to cook and have the ability to prepare simple, nutritious meals. Some people find cooking nutritious meals to be a difficult task. There are many meals in this book that can be prepared in twenty minutes or less. The recipes provided do not need to be followed exactly, rather they are more like a guide. Most ingredients can easily be substituted for other healthful ingredients in the same category if you do not like a particular item or you do not have it on hand.

Throughout this book you will learn about the following:
- Food safety

- How to properly store your food to maximize freshness and decrease spoilage
- How to be a savvy and health-conscious grocery store shopper
- How to decipher between nutritious foods and foods marketed as healthy foods
- How to cook recipes for commonly wasted

I highly recommend that everyone complete the kitchen cleanout, which is found in Chapter 4. Starting fresh and having an inventory of your ingredients sets the stage for future success.

If you want to learn how to prepare nutritious meals, save money at the grocery store, shop without being overwhelmed by nutrition claims and food marketing gimmicks, and store your food in ways that maximize freshness then this guidebook is for you.

## How to Use This Book

This book is written to be a guide for you to work through your kitchen struggles. Tips, exercises, and nutrition examples are provided to help you use the information to the best of your ability. Each chapter builds upon the next. While it would be beneficial to read this book from cover to cover, it is not necessary in the short term. This guidebook has clear and helpful chapters that will make it simple for you to find the section that best suits your needs. Think about what matters most to you. Do you want to start off with recipes? Do you struggle with keeping foods fresh?

The table of contents and index at the back of this book will help you to easily find the sections which you want to read/refer to.

# Chapter 2: Importance of Nutrition in the Kitchen

## Nutrition 101: Why You Should Care about What You Eat

The kitchen is where it all starts. It is where we cook, eat, gather, talk, and just hang around. In many households the kitchen is a source of family connection. What we produce there is not just a onetime meal, but an entire lifetime's worth of habits that shape our health and our family's health.

According to the Center for Disease Control, seven of the ten leading causes of death are diet and lifestyle related.[1] Diet and lifestyle-related diseases are in bold text.
1. **Heart disease**
2. **Cancer**
3. **Chronic lower respiratory disease**
4. Accidents
5. **Stroke**
6. **Alzheimer's disease**
7. **Diabetes**
8. Influenza and pneumonia
9. **Nephritis, nephrotic syndrome and nephrosis (kidney disease)**
10. Intentional self-harm (suicide)

The top three diseases on this list make up 50% of all deaths. As a registered dietitian, I have helped many people over the years create lifelong habits that improved their health. These changes were not drastic or time-consuming, but realistic and sustainable changes that fit into a busy lifestyle.

Simple daily tweaks to what you already do in the kitchen can greatly improve your health. Proper meal planning and reducing food waste will help you save money by lowering your grocery bill.

Think about these questions to help understand your eating/cooking habits. Do you cook? Do you heat up already prepared food such as frozen meals? Do you get takeout?

Here are some common reasons why people do not cook:
- It feels too difficult
- It takes too much time

- No one taught them how
- They never have the right ingredients

Below is an exercise to help you understand your habits and what changes will help you eat healthier and save money. Answer each question below either in the book or a separate piece of paper, then read below for tips that may improve your health.

---

Exercise: Understand your Eating Habits
1. How many unplanned trips do you make to the grocery store each week?
2. How many nights do you eat out or get takeout for dinner?
3. On average, how many food items do you throw away each week?
4. How often do you eat lunch out?
5. How many unplanned snacks do you purchase throughout the day?
6. How many ready-to-eat meals do you heat up each week?
7. How many times per week do you plan on cooking dinner at home but then order takeout?

---

The answers to the questions above should be closest to zero.

1. **How many unplanned trips do you make to the grocery store each week**?

   Unplanned grocery trips are an indication of poor grocery store shopping. You did not purchase enough food for the week to make well-balanced meals, did not know what foods to purchase initially, or you did not have a well-planned grocery list. Unplanned grocery trips lead to wasted time and unplanned spending. In the book *America's Cheapest Family*, "Shoppers making a 'quick trip' to the store to pick up a few specific items usually purchase 54% more than they planned."[2]

   To avoid unplanned trips to the grocery store, try planning your meals for the week and creating a shopping list based on your meal plan. See chapter 5 for a sample grocery list and meal plan. It is also important to learn how to substitute or omit ingredients in recipes. Most savory recipes do not need to be followed exactly. Chapter 7 lists common substitutions that can be made when cooking.

2. **How many nights do you eat out or get takeout for dinner?**

   Eating food away from home leads to consuming more calories, saturated fat, and added sugar than most home-cooked meals. Eating out frequently is also very costly. Even fast food, which most people think saves money, can become an expensive habit. See page 11 learn more about the costs of fast food.

According to a study from the *Journal of the Academy of Nutrition and Dietetics*, impulsivity (making decisions last minute) was associated with the frequency of fast-food consumption.[3] If you do not have a meal planned or prepped ahead of time, you will be more likely to grab food from a restaurant. Having a weekly meal plan will help you commit to making your meals at home.

Think about what gets in the way of cooking meals at home. Do you find cooking exhausting? Do you lack confidence in your cooking skills? Do you know how to prepare a well-balanced meal? See chapter 5 for information about meal planning and grocery shopping.

3. **On average, how many food items do you throw away each week?**

Food that is thrown out is a waste of money and has negative environmental implications or effects. Look at what you throw out and think about why.
   a. Did the food spoil because you forgot about it? If so, see chapter 4 to learn about proper placement of food in the refrigerator.
   b. Did the food spoil because you were not sure how to cook it? If so, see Chapter 7 for recipe ideas.
   c. Did you throw out leftovers? If so, take a look at table 3 on page 25 for uses for leftover ingredients.

4. **How often do you eat lunch out?**

Save lunches out for social occasions. Grabbing something to eat last minute at a fast food restaurant or in the cafeteria is an unnecessary cost and less healthful than packing a lunch from home. Leftovers are great for lunch. You can also prepare a week's worth of wraps, salads, or soups at the beginning of the week to save time. See chapter 5 on meal planning for ideas.

5. **How many unplanned snacks do you purchase throughout the day?**

Costs of snacks from vending machines or the convenience store have a large mark-up. Granola bars at a vending machine can cost as much as $1.50. If you purchase that granola bar five times per week, you will pay $7.50. For $7.50 you can purchase two dozen eggs that can be hardboiled, one pound of unsalted nuts, or even make an entire loaf of peanut butter and jelly sandwiches. All of these snacks can easily be prepared ahead of time.

6. **How many ready-to-eat meals do you heat up each week?**

Ready-to-eat meals are very high in sodium. See table 1 below for the health implications of sodium. Most people I talk to do not actually like already-prepared meals, but eat them because of convenience. Preparing part of your meals in advance will help reduce the time spent cooking dinner. See chapter 5 about meal planning.

7. **How many times per week do you plan on cooking dinner at home but then order takeout?**

Think about why you did not cook your planned meal. Did you run out of time? Not feel like cooking? Realize you did not have all the ingredients to make your dish? Try meal planning, learning some quick easy meals, and making the Crock-Pot your best friend.

# Cooking at Home: Your Wallet and Your Health

Cooking at home is one of the best things you can do for your health. A study by Johns Hopkins Bloomberg School of Public Health found that those who cook meals at home eat healthier and consume fewer calories than those who frequently ate out.[4] Restaurant food generally has more saturated fat, sodium, and added sugar than home-cooked meals. A study in the *Journal of the Academy of Nutrition and Dietetics* found that 92% of popular menu choices exceeded the recommended number of calories for a meal cooked at home[5] Once you start cooking more at home with nutritious ingredients, you will see improvements in your energy level, digestion, and general wellbeing. The table below explains how nutrients consumed in excess have a negative impact on your health.

| TABLE 1. Reference: Dietary Guidelines for Americans 2015 – 2020 | | |
|---|---|---|
| Nutrient | Health Implications | Foods |
| Saturated Fat / Trans Fat | Excessive amounts of saturated/trans fats increase your risk for developing cardiovascular disease. | Saturated fats and trans fats are found in fried foods, processed meats, and pastries, as well as mixed dishes containing cheese and/or meat, such as burgers, sandwiches, tacos and pizza. |
| Sodium | Sodium consumed in quantities greater than 2300 mg per day increase your risk for high blood | Sodium is found in processed foods such as canned soups, already-prepared frozen meals, fast food, condiments, and |

| | pressure and cardiovascular disease. | processed meats like bologna and sausage. |
|---|---|---|
| Added Sugars | Added sugars do not provide any essential nutrients. Instead, they increase your risk for type 2 diabetes, obesity, certain cancers, and cardiovascular disease | Added sugars are found in sweetened beverages, such as sodas, sweetened teas, and fruit-flavored drinks, pastries and syrups. Added sugars are frequently 'hidden' in foods such as cereals, granola bars, and condiments |

Often people think that fast food will save money, but this is not the case. A fast-food meal costs an average of $5 to $7 per meal per person. If you ate for all three meals, you would spend an average of $18 per day. For a family of four, this is an average of $72 for one day ($18/day x 4 people).[6] It will cost a family of four $168 per week if they eat dinner out every night of the week. With careful planning, you can purchase an entire week's worth of groceries for $168.

Learning how to be practical and resourceful in the kitchen is a great skill to have. This skill will help you and your family become healthier. Cooking at home can become a fun hobby and a great way to spend time together. It can also help you save money. Another way to save money is to handle your food properly and store it at the correct temperature. The next chapter focuses on food safety and will teach you how to safely handle food at home.

# Chapter 3: Food Safety 101

## Importance of Food Safety

Foodborne illness is a preventable health problem that is caused by food contaminated with bacteria, viruses, parasites, or toxins. The Federal Government estimates that there are 48 million cases of foodborne illness annually, which is the equivalent of sickening one in six Americans. Each year these cases result in an estimated 128,000 hospitalizations and 3,000 deaths.[7]

Once food reaches your home, it is important to handle it correctly. Learning how to handle food properly will not only keep you safe, it will also help preserve your food so it lasts longer. The refrigerator is one of the most important pieces of equipment in the kitchen for keeping food safe.

## Food Safety 101

One of the easiest ways to keep foods from spoiling is to keep them out of the temperature danger zone, which is 40°F to 140°F. Make sure to set the temperature in your refrigerator below 40°F and the temperature in your freezer at 0°F.

| ! Temperature Danger Zone ! |
|---|
| Bacteria, such as Salmonella, Staphylococcus aureus, and Escherichia coli (E. coli), grow most rapidly in the temperature range between 40°F and 140°F. This is called the temperature danger zone. You do not want to keep food in this temperature range for more than two cumulative hours. [8] |

### Check Your Refrigerator Temperature

Does your refrigerator have a built-in thermometer? Make sure it is reads 40°F or below. Temperatures above 40°F are in the temperature danger zone and put you at risk for many foodborne illnesses. If your refrigerator does not have a thermometer, consider buying one.

A survey showed that only 40% of people knew if their refrigerator was set at the right temperature (Zelman 2015).

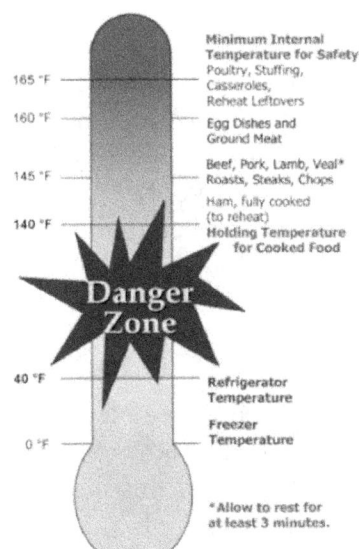

Try not to let foods remain in the temperature danger zone for more than two cumulative hours. This includes when letting cooked foods cool, after picking up food at the grocery store, and when defrosting. This can be challenging because food has to be transported home from the grocery store, usually via the car.

| Tip |
|---|
| When running errands, make grocery shopping your last trip. Remember to bring a hot/cold bag or a cooler to store your perishables on hot summer days. |

FIGURE 1. Food Safety
Inspection Service

## Clean, Separate, Cook, and Chill

The best way to prevent foodborne illnesses is to use the *Clean, Separate, Cook, and Chill* method.[9]

**Clean:** Wash your hands and cooking utensils thoroughly before cooking and after handling different foods, like meats and vegetables. Cross contamination is the transfer of harmful bacteria from one food to another food. It can happen when bacteria from foods like meat are passed to vegetables through unwashed hands, cutting boards, or utensils.[10]

**Separate:** Proper separation reduces the risk of cross contamination. When cooking, use separate cutting boards, utensils, and plates for produce, meat, poultry, and seafood. Separate these foods at the grocery store by placing meats and produce in different parts of your cart and bags when transporting. At home, place them on separate shelves in your refrigerator. The chart on page 20 shows you the proper placement of food in your refrigerator.

**Cook:** Use a food thermometer when cooking. Knowing the internal temperature of your food is the only way to ensure it is cooked properly. Food that is not cooked properly is at higher risk of developing foodborne illness. When reheating or microwaving food, cook to above 165°F.

**Chill:** Remember, foods should never be left in the temperature danger zone for more than two hours. Refrigerate perishable foods after two hours of cooking them. Defrosting, or thawing food safely is another important way to protect yourself against foodborne illness. The safest way to thaw food is by placing it on a plate on the bottom shelf of your refrigerator. The next safest way to thaw your food is to place it in an airtight bag then submerge the bag in cold water. Do not use hot or warm water, because hot water will start to cook your food. You can also thaw food in the microwave, but make sure to cook the food immediately.

Keep the temperature danger zone in mind when defrosting. Repeatedly thawing and refreezing food items will increase the amount of time they spend in the temperature danger zone. This puts your food at a higher risk for growing bacteria and becoming unsafe for consumption. The list below contains the safe ways to defrost food:

| ! Safe ways to defrost food ! |
| --- |
| 1.  In the refrigerator<br>2.  In cold water<br>3.  In the microwave |
| *Never defrost frozen food on the counter or in the sink. It will take much longer than two hours to completely defrost, thus making you very susceptible to a foodborne illness. |

## Reheating Leftovers Safely

Using leftovers is something I strongly advocate. Leftovers make quick meals and will save you money and keep food from entering the landfill. When reheating your leftovers, keep food safety in mind. Make sure the internal temperature of your meal reaches 165°F.[11]

Microwaves are frequently used to quickly heat up food. Unfortunately, they do not cook foods evenly. If you are using a microwave, place your food in a dish and add a small amount of liquid. The moisture will help destroy harmful bacteria and make sure the food cooks fully. Cover the dish with a loose-fitting lid before putting it in the microwave. Halfway through heating, stir the contents or flip the food over to make sure the entire contents reach 165°F.

Keeping your foods out of the temperature danger zone and handling them properly will keep you healthy by preventing foodborne illnesses. Having a well-organized kitchen and pantry will make it easier to prepare nutritious meals while reducing waste.

# Chapter 4: The Kitchen Cleanout

Now that you know the basics of food safety, it is time to go through your kitchen. Take this time to reflect on your habits that were discovered in exercise on page 8 and be mindful of patterns you see when going through your refrigerator and pantry.

## Why Do a Kitchen Cleanout?

A dirty refrigerator is a disaster waiting to happen for many reasons:
- A stuffed refrigerator is more likely to have a temperature in the temperature danger zone because there is less room for air to circulate.
- You are less likely to spot moldy food.
- It is difficult to know what you have on hand and what you might need. Unseen food items are more likely to be forgotten. That means lots of food waste and wasted money.

Think about your refrigerator. Is it so packed that you have trouble identifying what you have? Can you see any visibly spoiled foods? Is there a bad smell coming from somewhere? Are there any spills?

## Cleanout and Inventory

The first step in a refrigerator cleanout is to take everything out of the refrigerator. If your refrigerator is full, or a complete refrigerator cleanout feels overwhelming, consider working on one shelf at a time. Inspect each food item and determine the following:
- Is the product spoiled? If so, throw it out. This may be the only time you want to throw food away. But remember, you are starting fresh.
- Does it need to be consumed soon?
- Should it be re-packaged?
- Is it perfectly fine and maybe it was just forgotten?

| Indications of food spoilage |
|---|
| Mold, white fuzz, change in color, off odor, sliminess |

The next step in the kitchen cleanout is to create an inventory of what you have and what you need. Writing down all of the foods you have will help you understand your food-buying patterns. You will realize if you over-purchase, purchase the same items several times or foods that you purchase but never use. It will also help you determine what meals you can make with the food you have on hand.

The third step is to clean the refrigerator with some soap and warm water. If it has been a while since your refrigerator was cleaned, it may need a good scrubbing. Page 21 provides a recap of the kitchen cleanout steps for easy reference.

| Tip |
| --- |
| Hang a dry erase board on your refrigerator so you can write down the foods you have or foods you may forget to use. This is helpful when experimenting with new foods. Unfamiliar foods are more likely to be forgotten and as a result spoil. |

Now cleanout your pantry. Consolidate boxes of the same or similar food item and throw out/donate what you know you will not eat. Check with your local pantry for items that can and cannot be donated. Starting fresh will help you reduce food waste in the future.

| |
| --- |
| Visit the following sites to find a food pantry near you:<br>• http://ampleharvest.org/find-pantry/<br>• http://www.foodpantries.org |

# What Do the Expiration Dates Mean?

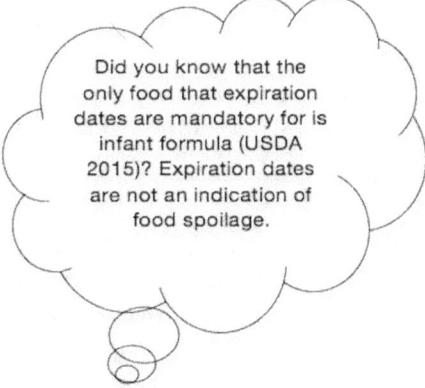

Did you know that the only food that expiration dates are mandatory for is infant formula (USDA 2015)? Expiration dates are not an indication of food spoilage.

When cleaning out your refrigerator, you may be inclined to use the expiration dates to determine whether an item has spoiled. These dates include Best if Used By, Sell By, Use By date. However, expiration dates are indication dates for best quality, not necessarily for safety.[12] The dates listed below are determined through storage studies or stability tests conducted by the product's manufacturer.[13] Remember these dates are only guidelines. If a food is handled improperly it will spoil before the expiration date; if a food is handled properly, it can last beyond the expiration dates.

You can use the dates listed on the package as a guide, but you do not need to depend on them to determine food spoilage. It is important to understand the dates listed, as there are several of them that can be confusing.

**Sell By Date**: This date is used by grocery stores to determine how long to display the product for sale.

**Best if Used By (or Best if Used Before)**: This date is recommended for best flavor or quality.

**Use By Date**: This date is the last date recommended for consumption of the product while at peak quality. Food can be safely consumed after this date if handled correctly.

# Placement of Food in the Refrigerator

Now that you have gone through all of your food, discarded or donated unwanted items, and taken an inventory of what you have, you need to put your food away. Placement of food in the refrigerator is key to keeping it fresh. Make sure not to overstuff your refrigerator. Packing the refrigerator with food will make it difficult for air to circulate, which can increase the temperature inside the refrigerator. When the temperature in the refrigerator increases, food spoils more quickly.[14]

The door shelves are best for foods that are less perishable, such as juice, butter, and condiments. This is the warmest part of the refrigerator. The upper shelves inside the refrigerator are best for more perishable foods, such as dairy products, eggs, leftovers, and already-cooked foods. The bottom shelves are the coldest part of the refrigerator and should be used for raw foods, such as meat, poultry, and fish.

| Tip |
|---|
| Raw meat and fish products should be sealed and placed on the bottom shelf. If they are on the top shelf, they can drip down and contaminate other foods. |

Use the crisper drawers for fruits and vegetables. Separate produce that produces ethylene from produce that is sensitive to ethylene. Ethylene is a plant hormone that triggers produce to degrade and to become overripe and eventually spoil.

| Table 2. List of Ethylene Producing and Ethylene Sensitive Fruit | |
| --- | --- |
| Ethylene-Producing Produce | Ethylene Sensitive Fruit |
| <ul><li>Stone fruits such as peaches and plums</li><li>Kiwis</li><li>Tomatoes</li><li>Apples and Pears</li><li>Avocados</li><li>Bananas</li><li>Cantaloupes</li><li>Melons</li></ul> | <ul><li>Asparagus</li><li>Broccoli</li><li>Carrots</li><li>Cucumbers</li><li>Eggplants</li><li>Green Beans</li><li>Lettuce and Leafy Greens</li><li>Potatoes</li><li>Summer Squash</li><li>Strawberries</li><li>Watermelons</li></ul> |

If you have a high-humidity drawer, place foods that tend to wilt and those that are sensitive to ethylene gas in that drawer. Foods that tend to rot or emit ethylene gas should be placed in the low-humidity drawer. Humidity drawers are also known as crispers. Some refrigerators will have a high and low setting that can be used to separate the ethylene producing produce from the produce sensitive to ethylene.

Note: Use the chart on the next page as a reference for proper food placement in the refrigerator.

# Proper Placement of Food in the Refrigerator

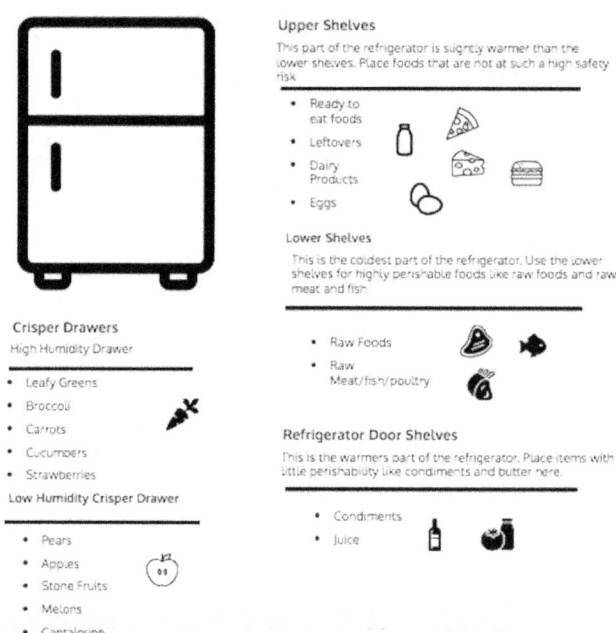

**Upper Shelves**

This part of the refrigerator is slightly warmer than the lower shelves. Place foods that are not at such a high safety risk.

- Ready to eat foods
- Leftovers
- Dairy Products
- Eggs

**Lower Shelves**

This is the coldest part of the refrigerator. Use the lower shelves for highly perishable foods like raw foods and raw meat and fish.

- Raw Foods
- Raw Meat/fish/poultry

**Refrigerator Door Shelves**

This is the warmer part of the refrigerator. Place items with little perishability like condiments and butter here.

- Condiments
- Juice

**Crisper Drawers**

High Humidity Drawer

- Leafy Greens
- Broccoli
- Carrots
- Cucumbers
- Strawberries

Low Humidity Crisper Drawer

- Pears
- Apples
- Stone Fruits
- Melons
- Cantaloupe

FIGURE 2. ADAPTED FROM FOOD SAFETY INSPECTION SERVICE

Now that you have cleaned out your refrigerator and pantry, keep it clean and organized. Keeping a clean refrigerator is key to improving your kitchen and your health.[15] If every time you open your refrigerator you get frustrated with not being able to find anything, or tired of seeing all of your fresh foods go bad, you will be less likely to want to cook. The environment of your kitchen plays a critical role in your health and motivation to cook.

| Tip |
| --- |
| You are more likely to grab foods that you see. Keep healthy foods in the front of your refrigerator or pantry. |

In the book *Does This Clutter Make My Butt Look Fat?*, Author Peter Walsh writes about the correlation between clutter (particularly kitchen clutter) and weight problems.[16] A cluttered kitchen gets in the way of healthful food preparation. Walsh gives the example of a dirty restaurant. You would not want to eat at a dirty, unorganized restaurant. This is also true for a home kitchen. The messier the kitchen, the less time you will want to spend time preparing healthy meals.

**Kitchen/Pantry Cleanout Recap**
1. Take everything out of your refrigerator/pantry
2. Inspect each item and determine which foods have spoiled and need to be tossed
3. Re-package foods if necessary
4. Write down what foods you have and distinguish between perishables and non-perishables
5. Wash your shelves with warm water and soap
6. Put foods back in their proper places *See figure 2

Have you bought groceries you did not mean to purchase? Did you know why these items ended up in your cart? The next chapter will help you navigate your way through the grocery store so this no longer happens.

# Chapter 5: Navigating the Grocery Store

## Creating a Personalized Grocery List

Did you know grocery stores contain over 42,000 food products?
[17] It is no wonder why so many of us leave with food items we do not need, or missing the items we meant to purchase. This is why lists are so important. When you become distracted by all the items on the shelf, the list will help you remember what you really need to buy. However, writing a list is not as simple as it sounds. It requires planning.

I have spoken to many clients who struggled to create grocery lists that could get them through the week without needing to purchase food last minute or wasting food due to poor planning. Creating a successful grocery list takes time. You need to understand your habits, food preferences, and nutritional needs. You should only need to shop once per week, unless you buy your produce at a farmers' market that is only open one day of the week, or you pick up meats at your favorite butcher on your way home from work. If you shop at one store for all your groceries, aim for one shopping trip per week. Avoiding last minute grocery trips will greatly reduce your grocery bill.

### Step One: Deciding What You Like

When I help clients make personalized grocery lists, I like to have them divide ingredients into food groups. By basing meals on food groups, you ensure that you have a nutritious meal.

A nutritious meal is a well-balanced meal that includes complex carbohydrates, lean proteins, healthy fats, and as many nonstarchy vegetables as you can.

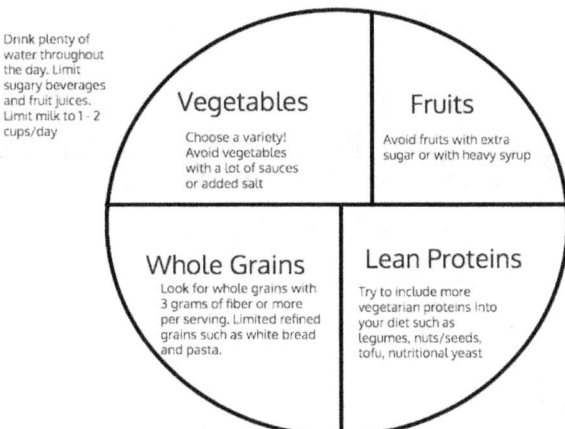

FIGURE 3. Adapted from Harvard School of Public Health

Below is a list of foods that will help guide you when making a meal.

| TABLE 2. Nutritious Foods Based on Food Group/Category (Dietary Guidelines 2015) |
| --- |
| List of Healthy Fats <br> • Olive Oil <br> • Nuts and Seeds <br> • Fatty Fish (Salmon, Tuna, Trout, Herring, Sardines, Mackerel) <br> • Avocado |
| List of Healthy/Complex Carbohydrates <br> • Starchy Vegetables (Potatoes with Skin, Corn, Peas, Winter Squash) <br> • Whole Grains (See page 30 <br> • Beans |
| List of Lean Proteins <br> • Beans <br> • Plain Yogurt <br> • Milk/Soy Milk <br> • Nuts and Seeds <br> • Eggs <br> • Baked/Broiled Chicken or Fish <br> • Lean Red Meat <br> • Tofu <br> • Nutritional Yeast |

Using the information listed in table above choose at least seven healthy carbohydrate foods and seven healthy protein foods that you like and would enjoy eating for dinner. Then think of what non-starchy vegetables (any vegetable except for potatoes, peas, corn and winter squash) you would like to have with dinner. Make sure to use perishable carbohydrates such as already cooked rice and proteins, like dairy meat, or fish, at the beginning of the week.

| Tip |
|---|
| If by mid-week you decide not to use a perishable protein, such as meat, chicken or fish, freeze it. Once it has been safely defrosted, you can cook it like you purchased it fresh. |

## Step Two: Creating the List

Before grocery shopping, check your home inventory to see what you already have. Knowing what you already have will help you save money by purchasing fewer food items. Next, think about what you can make with your ingredients. Do you have leftover vegetables? Plan on making soup. Consider what other ingredients you will need to make the soup. Do you have these ingredients? Do you need to purchase them? Consider the other foods you have on hand. If they are perishable, figure out how you can incorporate them into the next two meals. Read chapter 7 and/or table 3 for meal ideas and leftovers perishables.

Leftovers can include any food that you did not use. It can be single ingredients, like spinach, or plain pasta, or part of an already-cooked meal, such as roasted chicken. As long as the ingredient or meal did not spoil, it can be used in another dish. It is best to use already-cooked foods first as they will spoil faster than foods that have not been cooked.

| Table 3. Making meals with Leftover Ingredients * Recipes in Chapter 7 | | |
|---|---|---|
| **Ingredients You Have** | **What You Can Make** | **What You Need** |
| Protein (Chicken, Beans, Meat, Nuts and Seeds) | Rice Bowl | Rice, Vegetables, Salsa/Sauce |
| | Soup | Vegetables, Broth/Stock or Water, Starch |
| | Fajitas/Tacos | Tortillas, Vegetables, Salsa/Dressing |
| | Nut Parfait or Oatmeal Bowl | Oats, Yogurt, Milk, Fruit |
| Nonstarchy vegetables | Soup | Protein, Broth/Stock, Grains/Potatoes |
| | Casserole/Frittata | Eggs, Grains (Quinoa, Rice, Potatoes), Cheese, Milk, Herbs/Spices |
| Carbohydrates (Leftover Rice, Pasta, Potatoes, Corn or Peas) | Rice bowl | Protein, Vegetables, Salsa/Sauce |
| | Soups | Protein, Vegetables, Broth/Water, Herbs |
| | Frittata | Eggs, Vegetables |
| | Pasta Bowl | Protein, Vegetables, Sauce/Sauce |

| TABLE 4. Weekly Menu for Two Adults *Recipes in Chapter 7 | | | | | | |
|---|---|---|---|---|---|---|
| | **Monday** | **Tuesday** | **Wednesday** | **Thursday** | **Friday** | **Saturday** |
| Breakfast | Yogurt Parfait | Yogurt Parfait | Overnight Oats | Overnight Oats | Egg and Spinach Sandwich | Egg and Spinach Sandwich |
| Lunch | Nut Butter Sandwich | Leftovers | Leftovers | Leftovers | Leftovers | Leftovers |
| Dinner (See chapter 7 for recipes) | Beef and Lentil Stew | Salmon Fajitas | Whole Roasted Chicken with Potatoes and brussels sprouts | Stuffed Peppers | Zucchini Cakes with Quinoa | Rice Bowl with Leftover Ingredients |
| Snacks | Hard-Boiled Eggs, Hummus and Vegetables, Nut Butter and Apples | | | | | |

| TABLE 5. Grocery List For Two Adults |
| --- |
| **Dry Goods** |
| ☐  2 cups rice/2.5 lbs. |
| ☐  1 package whole wheat tortillas |
| ☐ 3 cups rolled oats/1-18oz package |
| ☐ 1 28-oz. can crushed tomatoes |
| ☐ 1 cup lentils/1 lb. |
| ☐ 1 cup quinoa /1 lb. |
| ☐ 1 cup whole wheat flour/0.5 lb. |
| **Meats/Fish/Cheese/Eggs** |
| ☐ 1 lb. ground beef |
| ☐ 1 whole chicken |
| ☐ 1 14-oz. can of canned salmon |
| ☐ 1 block sharp cheddar cheese (around 8 ounces) |
| ☐ 1 dozen eggs |
| **Other** |
| ☐  16 oz. hummus |
| **Dairy Products** |
| ☐ 1-32 ounce container of plain yogurt |
| ☐ ½ - 1 gallon of milk of choice (depends if you need it for coffee) |
| **Condiments/Spices** |
| ☐  1-15.5 oz. nut butter of choice |
| ☐  1-16 oz. bottle olive oil |
| ☐  salt |
| ☐  pepper |
| ☐  garlic powder |
| **Fruits/Vegetables** |
| ☐ 1 lime |
| ☐ 1 lemon |
| ☐ 1 avocado |
| ☐ 1 bag carrots |
| ☐ 1 lb. spinach |
| ☐ 2 onions |
| ☐ 4 apples |
| ☐ 1 lb. arugula |
| ☐ 4 medium potatoes |
| ☐ 1 lb. brussels sprouts |
| ☐ 1 garlic bulb |
| ☐ 2 medium zucchini |
| ☐ 2 cups fresh fruit of choice for oatmeal |

This may seem like a lot of groceries, but remember to check your pantry first. You may have some of the items, like dry goods and condiments, on hand.

| Tip |
|---|
| If you frequently throw away fresh produce, try frozen. Sometimes frozen produce is healthier than fresh. Some fresh produce may be wilted or have a lack of color. In this case frozen produce may be the better choice. If your fruits and vegetables end up in the trash, you are not getting any nutrition from them. Start with a few frozen vegetables to get into the habit of eating vegetables with each meal. After you get the hang of routinely incorporating frozen vegetables into your meals, start purchasing limited quantities of fresh produce and add them to your meals. Pay attention to how well you are using your fresh produce. The more you use it, the easier it will be to cook with. Chapter 7 has more information about getting started with frozen produce. |

# Alternative Grocery Shopping

Grocery stores are not the only place to purchase food. Farmers' markets and Community Supported Agriculture (CSA) are great ways to get healthy produce and other ingredients while supporting your local economy and small farmers. Farmers' markets and CSAs sell seasonal produce that has not traveled very far. Eating locally and seasonally is tastier, fresher, and better for the environment than produce that has traveled a long distance.

At farmers' markets, the farmers are often eager to talk about their produce. Often they will suggest ways to cook with it and might even allow you to try it. By getting to know your local farmers, you will become more appreciative of your food and take pride in what you eat. Farmers will talk to you honestly about how they grow their foods and any inputs such as fertilizer or pesticides/herbicides that they use. Farmers' markets are also great social events. Some farmers' markets have live music and food demonstrations.

Community Supported Agriculture is a system where you purchase a share of the farmer's crop before the season starts. This share typically provides you with a weekly box of produce. Shares vary in cost and the quantity of produce available. Some shares may include dairy products, meats, and eggs. Some CSAs allow you to select the produce you wish to receive; however, often you can easily swap with other members of the CSA if you receive something you do not like. Purchasing shares helps farmers with their costs at the beginning of the season and helps them pay for inputs, such as seeds and equipment.

**Tips for Shopping at a Farmers' Market**
- Bring cash as many markets are cash only.
- Walk around the market first to get an idea of what is available.
- If a food item is unfamiliar, do not be afraid to ask how to use it.

- If you need a large quantity of a specific item, ask if the farmer offers any discounts for bulk purchases.
- Bring your own bag.
- Bring an umbrella. Farmers' markets run rain or shine!

**Tips for Signing up for a CSA**

- Figure out your budget.
- Ask what produce the farmer intends to grow to ensure you will like most of what you will receive in your share.
- Know when you will be out of town, as pickups are often weekly. Do not let this deter you though, some CSAs are flexible.
- Learn about the farm and the farmer. Make sure you believe in the farm's practices.

---

Visit the following site to find farmer's markets and CSAs near you:
- www.localhavest.org

---

# Marketing Gimmicks and Food Label Confusion

Out of the 42,000 products found in the average grocery store, most are unhealthy and more expensive than the foods needed for a healthy diet. Food marketers are very good at their jobs. They want you to purchase their food products, especially the processed ones that are full of refined carbohydrates and cheap sugars. Learning about marketing gimmicks will help you be a savvy shopper and purchase the most healthful foods.

| Tip |
| --- |
| The best way to determine if a food product is healthy is to look at the ingredients and nutrition facts label. Remember ingredients are listed in order from the largest quantity to lowest quantity that is present in the food. |

### Natural

The term natural has no regulation for its use. The Food and Drug Administration has not developed a definition for the use of the term natural or its derivatives.[18] This means that food companies can decide to put the label *natural* on their products without adhering to any regulations. According to the senior scientists at the Environmental Working Group, there is not much difference between artificial flavor and natural flavor.[19] In fact there is no definition for the term 'natural'. See the example below.

## Regular Cheetos

**Nutrition Facts**

Serving Size 1 oz

**Amount Per Serving**

**Calories** 150          Calories from Fat 90

|  | % Daily Values* |
| --- | --- |
| **Total Fat** 10g | **15%** |
| Saturated Fat 1.5g | **8%** |
| Trans Fat 0g | |
| **Sodium** 300mg | **13%** |
| **Total Carbohydrate** 13g | **4%** |
| Dietary Fiber 0g | **0%** |
| Sugars 1g | |
| **Protein** 2g | **4%** |

* Percent Daily Values are based on a 2,000 calorie diet.

## Natural Cheetos

**Nutrition Facts**

Serving Size 1 oz

**Amount Per Serving**

**Calories** 150          Calories from Fat 80

|  | % Daily Values* |
| --- | --- |
| **Total Fat** 9g | **14%** |
| Saturated Fat 1.5g | **8%** |
| Trans Fat 0g | |
| **Sodium** 290mg | **12%** |
| **Total Carbohydrate** 16g | **5%** |
| Dietary Fiber 0g | **0%** |
| Sugars 1g | |
| **Protein** 2g | **4%** |

* Percent Daily Values are based on a 2,000 calorie diet.

**Cheetos Puffs (Made with Real Cheese)**

Ingredients

Enriched Corn Meal (Corn Meal, ferrous Sulfate, Niacin, Thiamin Mononitrate, Riboflavin and Folic Acid), Vegetable Oil (Corn, Canola, and/or Sunflower Oil), Cheese Seasoning (Whey, Cheddar Cheese [Milk, Cheese Cultures, Salt, Enzymes], Canola Oil, Maltodextrin [Made from Corn], Salt, Whey Protein Concentrate, Monosodium Glutamate, Natural and Artificial Flavors, Lactic Acid, Citric Acid, Artificial Color (Yellow 6) and Salt

**Simply Cheetos Puffs (Made with Real Cheese)**

Ingredients

Organic Corn Meal, Expeller-Pressed Sunflower Oil, Whey, Cheddar Cheese (Milk, Cheese Cultures, Salt, Enzymes), Maltodextrin (Made from Corn), Sea Salt, Natural Flavors, Sour Cream (Cultured Cream, Skim Milk), Torula Yeast, Lactic Acid and Citric Acid.

FIGURE 4. FRITO LAY 2016.

The label to the right is a *natural* version of Cheetos, and the one to the left is their regular version. When looking at the packages at the grocery store, you may think that the natural version is healthier. But, if you examine the nutrition facts label, you will notice that they have the same number of calories per serving. Sure, there are fewer ingredients in the natural version, but one of the ingredients is *natural flavors*, which again has no definition.

## Multigrains Versus Whole Grains

Whole grains contain all parts of the kernel, includes the bran, endosperm, and germ. Processed or refining the grain normally removes the bran and the germ, leaving only the endosperm. When the bran and germ are removed, 25% of a grain's protein is lost along with seventeen key nutrients.[20]

Products labeled as multigrain contain more than one type of grain. But that does not mean all of the grains listed in the ingredients are whole grains. Below is a list of whole grains.

| TABLE 7. Types of Whole Grains |
| --- |
| Amaranth |
| Barley |
| Buckwheat |
| Corn (Includes Whole Cornmeal and Popcorn) |
| Millet |
| Oats (Includes Oatmeal) |
| Quinoa |
| Rice (Includes Brown and Colored Rice) |
| Rye |
| Sorghum (Also Called Milo) |
| Teff |
| Triticale |
| Wheat (Includes Varieties such as Spelt, Emmer, Farro, Einkorn, Kamut, Durum and Forms such as Bulgur, Cracked Wheat and Wheat Berries Wild Rice) |

Another common confusion is the difference between whole grain and whole wheat. Wheat is a type of grain. All whole wheat is whole grain, but not all whole grains are whole wheat.

Consider the organic multigrain pretzels listed below. The first ingredient is organic wheat flour. It does not say *whole* wheat flour, or 100% *whole wheat*, so you cannot be completely sure if the produce is actually whole wheat. If you look towards the bottom of the food label, you will see whole oat flour. Because there are two different types of grains (wheat and oats) this product can be labeled multigrain.

| Organic Multigrain Pretzel Rings |
| --- |
| Ingredients |
| Organic wheat flour, organic vegetable oil (contains organic expeller pressed sunflower oil and organic palm fruit shortening), organic evaporated cane syrup, organic whole oat flour |

The best way to make sure you are purchasing a whole grain is to look at the ingredients. The first ingredient should be a whole grain, such as whole wheat, whole oats, or one of the grains listed below.

All whole grains are nutritious. They are a good source of fiber and many vitamins and minerals. Some of these grains, such as teff or kamut, may be unfamiliar to you. Many of these grains can be purchased at health food stores and co-ops. The good news is that many of these grains are becoming more well-known and are appearing at conventional grocery stores.

| To learn how to prepare whole grains visit the Whole Grains Council website: <br> • http://wholegrainscouncil.org/recipes/cooking-whole-grains |
| --- |

## Reduced

The term reduced means 25% less than the original product.[21] For example, a box of cookies labeled as *reduced sugar* has 25% less sugar than the original product. However, this does not mean that the cookies are healthy. If the original box of cookies contain 100 grams of sugar per serving, then the reduced cookies contain 75 grams of sugar which is still a lot of sugar. Do not be fooled.

## Pringles Original

**Nutrition Facts**

Serving Size 1 oz

**Amount Per Serving**

**Calories** 150          Calories from Fat 90

% Daily Values*

| | |
|---|---|
| **Total Fat** 9g | **14%** |
| Saturated Fat 2.5g | **13%** |
| Trans Fat 0g | |
| **Sodium** 150mg | **6%** |
| **Total Carbohydrate** 15g | **5%** |
| Dietary Fiber 1g | **4%** |
| Sugars 0g | |
| **Protein** 1g | **2%** |

*Percent Daily Values are based on a 2,000 calorie diet.

## Pringles Reduced Fat

**Nutrition Facts**

Serving Size 1 oz

**Amount Per Serving**

**Calories** 140          Calories from Fat 70

% Daily Values*

| | |
|---|---|
| **Total Fat** 7g | **11%** |
| Saturated Fat 2g | **10%** |
| Trans Fat 0g | |
| **Sodium** 135mg | **6%** |
| **Total Carbohydrate** 17g | **6%** |
| Dietary Fiber 1g | **4%** |
| Sugars 0g | |
| **Protein** 1g | **2%** |

*Percent Daily Values are based on a 2,000 calorie diet.

FIGURE 5. Frito Lay

Take these Pringles® for example. The one on the right is the reduced-fat version, which contains 25% less fat than the 9 grams of fat in the original. Seven grams of fat is a lot for a snack. If you compare the total calories you will see that the reduced-fat version contains 10 fewer calories than the original version. This is because the reduced-fat version has more carbohydrates. Manufactures will often add more sugar to fat-free products and more fat to sugar-free products to compensate for taste. As a result many reduced-fat and reduced-sugar products have a similar number of calories as the original version. Unfortunately, most reduced products are not healthy choices.

## Good Source of ....

The claim "Good source of" means the product contains 10% or more of the Percent Daily Value (% DV) of a nutrient in one serving of food.[22] You have probably seen "Good Source of Fiber," "Good Source of Vitamin C," and "Good Source of Iron" on food packaging. Generally, it is good when a food has a good source of a healthy nutrient. However, many foods that are good sources of vitamin C or fiber are not very healthy due to high amounts of other unhealthful ingredients. Take this box of Froot Loops for example. On the top of the box it says "Good Source of Fiber."

| Kellogg's Froot Loops |
| --- |
| "Good Source of Fiber & Made with Whole Grains" |
| Ingredients |
| Sugar, corn flour blend (whole grain yellow corn flour, degerminated yellow corn flour), wheat flour, whole grain oat flour, oat fiber, modified food starch, soluble corn fiber, contains 2% or less of hydrogenated vegetable oil (coconut, soybean, and/or cottonseed), salt, natural flavor, red 40, turmeric extract color, yellow 6, blue 1, annatto extract color, BHT for freshness. |

Did you notice that the first ingredient on the label is sugar? This means that out of all the ingredients listed, this food product contains mostly sugar. Even though Froot Loops contain 3 grams of fiber per serving, this cereal is not a health food.

The American Heart Association (AHA) recommends limiting the amount of added sugars you consume to no more than half of your daily discretionary calories allowance. Discretionary calories are those that do not have a lot of vitamins and minerals, and therefore should be kept to a minimum. For most American women, that is no more than 100 calories per day, or about 6 teaspoons or 25 grams of sugar. For men, it is 150 calories or about 9 teaspoons of sugar or 37 grams of sugar per day. There are 4 calories per gram of sugar.[23]

## Made with Real Fruit

Real fruit is great, right? Fruit is full of fiber, vitamins, and minerals. Often when we hear that something is made with real fruit, we tend to think of it as a healthful food since fruit is a natural food. However this is not the case with many products containing the label "Made with real fruit."

**Outshine Fruit Bars: Mango**

**Nutrition Facts**

Serving Size 1 bar

**Amount Per Serving**

**Calories** 80

| | % Daily Values* |
|---|---|
| **Total Fat** 0g | 0% |
| Saturated Fat 0g | 0% |
| Trans Fat 0g | |
| **Cholesterol** 0mg | 0% |
| **Sodium** 0mg | 0% |
| **Total Carbohydrate** 20g | 7% |
| Dietary Fiber 0g | 0% |
| Sugars 19g | |
| **Protein** 0g | 0% |

Vitamin A 2%  •  Vitamin C 20%

*Percent Daily Values are based on a 2,000 calorie diet. Your Daily Values may be higher or lower depending on your calorie needs.

| | Calories | 2,000 | 2,500 |
|---|---|---|---|
| Total Fat | Less than | 65g | 80g |
| Sat Fat | Less than | 20g | 25g |
| Cholesterol | Less than | 300mg | 300mg |
| Sodium | Less than | 2400mg | 2400mg |
| Total Carbohydrate | | 300g | 375g |
| Dietary Fiber | | 25g | 30g |

| Outshine Fruit Bars Mango |
|---|
| Ingredients |
| Mango Puree, Water, Mango Juice from Concentrate, Cane Sugar, Lemon Juice, Natural Flavor, Guar Gum, Carob Bean Gum, Ascorbic Acid |

FIGURE 6. Outshine

Did you notice that the fourth ingredient is added sugar? Real fruit does not contain any added sugars. It does, however, contain fiber. The Outshine Fruit Bars pictured in figure 3 do not have any fiber. The term made with real fruit does not tell you how much fruit is actually in the product. Often times (like this product) 'real fruit' is not the first ingredient, or even the second.

## Now with No High Fructose Corn Syrup

High fructose corn syrup is a sugar that has been attributed to health conditions like cardiovascular disease, obesity, and type 2 diabetes. Many food companies are marketing their beverages with the claim "Now with No High Fructose Corn Syrup."

However, just because a beverage or food item no longer contains high fructose corn syrup, does not mean it is free of added sugar. Added sugar has been linked to the same health adversities as high fructose corn syrup (HFCS).

| Capri Sun (Now with no High Fructose Corn Syrup) |
|---|
| Ingredients |
| Filtered water, sugar, pear and grape juice concentrates, citric acid, orange, apple, and pineapple juice concentrates, natural flavor |

## Nutrition Facts

Serving Size 1 pouch

**Amount Per Serving**

**Calories** 50

| | % Daily Values* |
|---|---|
| **Total Fat** 0g | 0% |
| Saturated Fat 0g | 0% |
| Trans Fat 0g | |
| **Sodium** 15mg | 1% |
| **Total Carbohydrate** 14g | 5% |
| Dietary Fiber 0g | 0% |
| Sugars 13g | |
| **Protein** 0g | 0% |

*Percent Daily Values are based on a 2,000 calorie diet.

FIGURE 7. Capri Sun

Capri Sun has no artificial colors, flavors, preservatives, or high fructose corn syrup. This information is added to the label to get the consumer to believe Capri Sun is a healthy choice. However, when looking closely at the ingredients you will see that the second ingredient is still sugar. This is added sugar. No matter what the label says it does not contain, this beverage still is not a healthy choice. It does not provide any nutrition.

Sugary beverages increase the risk of type 2 diabetes, heart disease, and other chronic conditions. Those who regularly consume sugary drinks (one 12-oz.) have a 26% greater risk of developing type 2 diabetes than those who rarely consume sugary beverages. [24]

The reason to discuss marketing schemes is to make you aware of all the ploys food manufacturers use to encourage shoppers to purchase their products. Many of the food items marketed as healthy are a waste of money, and not needed in a healthy diet.

| Instead of | Do This |
|---|---|
| Purchasing a $5 box of sugary cereal advertised as healthy that will leave you hungry an hour later… | Make a high protein oatmeal bowl that will leave you satisfied for several hours. Soak ½ cup of oats in milk overnight. The next morning top with yogurt, nuts or seeds, and fruit. |
| Purchasing a fruit bar that has a lot of added sugars…… | Mix frozen fruit and a can of coconut milk or yogurt in a high-power blender. |

# The Grocery Store Maze

The grocery store is designed to encourage you to purchase more food than you wanted and intended. According to consumer expert Paco Underhill, "We had no intention of buying two thirds of what we buy in the supermarket."[25]

Placement of food items, lighting, and even music are purposefully designed to get consumers to spend more time and more money in the grocery store. According to a study conducted by Bangor University, after forty minutes of total shopping, many people are unable to shop practically and start shopping emotionally. Fifty percent of unintended purchases are the result of emotional shopping.[26] If you have been running errands all day, and the grocery store is the last stop, there is a high probability that you are shopping emotionally.

Grocery stores want you to shop with your stomach rather than your head.[27] Common staples most shoppers purchase on a regular basis, like eggs, butter, cheese, and milk, are located in the back of the store. This forces shoppers to pass aisles and displays that will entice them to purchase more food than intended. Specifically, the grocery store displays foods that will stimulate your senses like baked goods, fresh produce, and flowers near the entrance. Often the first display shoppers see when entering a grocery store is the produce department. It is believed that when people put fresh produce in their cart first, they feel better about themselves for making healthy choices. These positive feelings can lead shoppers to indulge in unhealthy food purchases towards the end of their shopping.

Take notice of the size of your grocery cart. It has gotten much bigger over the last several years. A larger cart encourages you to purchase more food even when you were not planning on doing so.

Grocery stores charge food companies slotting fees to place their products on store shelves. Since shoppers tend to see and purchase foods at eye level, products placed at eye level are the most expensive. The companies that can afford to pay these high slotting fees are usually big companies that have a lot of money and are not necessarily selling healthy products.[28] Look at the bottom shelf before automatically picking up what you see on an eye-level shelf.

The food products that you usually see on the end of the aisles are often convenience foods like sodas and snacks.[29] These products are frequently unhealthy and lead to unplanned purchases that provide a high profit margin to the retailer.

## Coupons: Do They Really Help You?

Coupons can save money if you use them correctly. Many shoppers clip coupons and feel compelled to use them.[30] You might save $0.50 on an item, but would you have purchased that item if you did not have the coupon? Many coupons force you to purchase two of an item in order to redeem the coupon, when you would normally purchase one product, or maybe none at all. One of the biggest reasons for spending too much money at the grocery store, and wasting food, is purchasing unnecessary items or larger quantities than you can use.

| Tip |
|---|
| Do not be tempted to purchase foods that you would not normally buy, just because you have a coupon. Using the coupon just to use it will not save you money. |

Everyone wants to spend less money at the grocery store. Many shoppers look at the sales circular when they first walk into the store. While the circular will list the sales for the week, it may not list the most healthful food items. A study conducted by the Academy of Nutrition and Dietetics evaluated one year of sales circulars and found that most circulars advertised unhealthful foods. Vegetables and fruits were advertised the least, while foods high salt and empty calories were the most advertised items.[31] Refrain from purchasing foods just because they are on sale or using the sales circulator as the basis for your grocery list. Write your list first then see if any of the foods you would like to purchase are in the sales circular or select an alternative brand or food similar to what you intended to purchase.

Everyone would like to spend less money on their grocery bill. A key way to save money on your groceries is to waste less food. Wasting food is equal to wasting money. The next chapter highlights the economic impact of food waste.

# Chapter 6: Economic Impact of Food Waste

According to Secretary of Agriculture Tom Vilsack, "An average family of four leaves more than two million calories of food, worth nearly $1,500, uneaten each year."[32] To break this down further, that is $125 each month and $31 each week in wasted food. Think about what you could do with the average $1,500 per year that is wasted due to food waste?

To give you a clearer picture of this waste, consider the following example. The average cost of a whole chicken is $1.50 per pound. A family of four wastes 200 5-lb. chickens per year. That is 16 5-lb. chickens each month or 4 5-lb. chickens each week.

That is a lot of wasted money! Some of you reading this book may be wasting even more money.

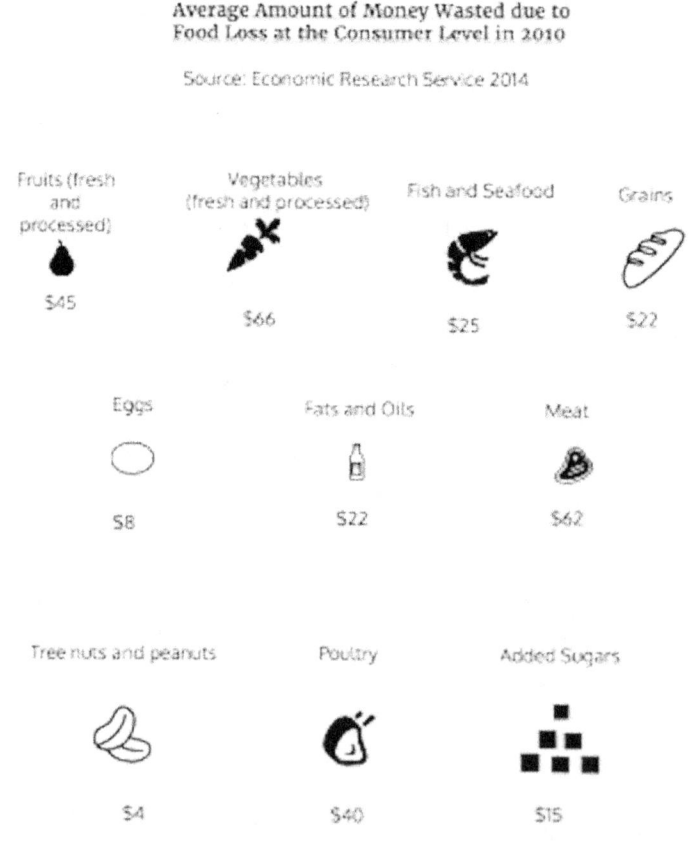

Average Amount of Money Wasted due to
Food Loss at the Consumer Level in 2010

Source: Economic Research Service 2014

| Fruits (fresh and processed) | Vegetables (fresh and processed) | Fish and Seafood | Grains |
|---|---|---|---|
| $45 | $66 | $25 | $22 |

| Eggs | Fats and Oils | Meat |
|---|---|---|
| $8 | $22 | $62 |

| Tree nuts and peanuts | Poultry | Added Sugars |
|---|---|---|
| $4 | $40 | $15 |

FIGURE 8. Economic Research Service

You can save money and help protect the environment by decreasing food waste at home. The earlier chapters provided strategies and tips to help decrease food waste through proper food handling and food safety. The next chapter provides guides and tips for optimizing food storage, instructions for long-term food preservation, recipes, and cooking tips.

# Chapter 7: Storage, Cooking Tips, and Recipes

This chapter ties all the previous chapters together. Now that you have learned about food safety, how to navigate the grocery store, and what constitutes a well-balanced meal, you are ready to start cooking. The recipes provided in this chapter require less than twenty minutes of active/prep-time time and do not involve many ingredients. It is not necessary to follow the recipes exactly, although you may want to do this when you first prepare these meals, especially if cooking is new to you. Ingredients, especially vegetables, can be substituted or even omitted. As long as you use another ingredient in the same category (such as substituting rice for quinoa or pasta), the dish will be tasty. See table 9 on page 49 for common substitutions you can use while cooking. Storage instructions are listed by specific food items.

## Meal Prep and Snacks

Meal prepping can save you a lot of time, money, and wasted calories. It will also reduce the amount of food you waste at home. Throwing together a last-minute meal is much easier when some of the ingredients are already chopped and pre-cooked. You are more likely to include vegetables in your meals when they are already precut or cooked. Meal prepping not only helps with last minute dinners, but it also helps with having healthy snacks on hand. Snacking is one of America's favorite pastimes. National dietary surveys have found that 90% of adults, 83% of adolescents, and 97% of children snack every day.[33] According to What We Eat in America's (WWEIA) 2007 – 2008 survey, foods and beverages consumed as snacks contribute an average of 586 calories for men and 421 calories for women.[34] This is roughly 20%-40% of our recommended daily intake.

Snacks can definitely be part of a healthy diet, but more often they wind up being added calories that do not contribute much nutrition to the diet. According to WWEIA the top five most consumed snacks are alcoholic beverages, sugar-sweetened beverages, salty snacks like pretzels, tortilla, potato chips, crackers, and sweet snacks such as candies and cakes, pastries and pies.

The table below provides examples of foods that can be prepared ahead of time to create a quick meal or snack.

| Table 8. List of foods that can be prepared ahead of time | | |
|---|---|---|
| Food | How to Prep | Uses |
| Chopped Vegetables (Carrots, Peppers, Onions, and Celery) | Wash and slice vegetables. Place them in airtight containers and store in the refrigerator. | Snacks, Sautés, Any Cooked Dish |
| Chicken | Grill, Roast or Bake | Topping for Salads, Tacos/Burritos, Rice Bowls, Pasta Dishes |
| Pre-Cooked Rice | Cook rice according to package directions. Place in airtight containers and store in the refrigerator. | Rice Bowls, Soups, Frittatas |
| Hard-Boiled Eggs | Store hard-boiled eggs in the refrigerator. You do not need to peel them right away. Hard-boiled eggs are actually easier to peel when the eggs have been in the refrigerator for several hours. | Snacks, Salad Topping, Egg Salad |
| Leafy Greens | Wash and chop dark leafy greens. Let the greens air dry as much as possible or place them in a salad spinner. Store greens in the refrigerator. | Salads, Quick Omelets, Sautés |
| Pre-Cooked Beans | Soak beans overnight. Rinse the beans and add new water to a stockpot. Cover and bring beans to a boil. Cook the beans for 45-90 minutes, depending on the type of bean. | Salad Topping, Rice Bowls |

# Leftover Ingredient Recipes

Using leftover ingredients is a great way to save money on your grocery bill and decrease food waste. Leftover meals, or leftover ingredients, can be incorporated into other dishes.

The recipes below provide guidelines for preparing simple meals that use leftover ingredients.

One of my favorite meals to cook is pizza. Pizza can be a great addition to your weekly meals if you use nutritious ingredients. Whole-wheat pizza dough is a great way to add whole grains and fiber to your diet. Almost any vegetable tastes good on pizza topped with cheese. Vegetable pizza is a great way to get vegetables in to your diet. It is also a fun meal to make with kids. Do not be afraid of working with flour and yeast. You do not have to be a skilled baker to make pizza dough from scratch. Try this simple recipe below.

| Whole Wheat Pizza Dough (Makes Two Loaves) |
|---|
| • 2 cups whole wheat flour<br>• 1 cup room-temperature water<br>• 1 ¼-oz. package instant yeast<br>• ½ teaspoon salt<br>• 1 teaspoon of herb such as oregano, thyme, rosemary, etc.<br>In a large bowl mix the flour, salt, herbs and instant yeast. Add the water and let it sit for 5 minutes until the mixture is foamy. In a stand mixer or a food processor, mix with the paddle attachment or dough blade for 2 – 3 minutes. If you do not have a stand mixer or a food processor knead with your hands for about 7 minutes. Cover bowl with a towel and let it sit for at least 2 hours. I like to make my pizza dough before work and leave it for 8 hours.<br><br>Cut the dough in half and let it sit for 5 minutes. Flour a surface and roll out dough. If you only want to make one pizza, wrap the other loaf in plastic wrap and place it in the freezer. To defrost the pizza dough, place it in the refrigerator the night before you want to use it.<br><br>To use the dough simply roll out on a floured surface until about ½ inch thick. Add sauce, cheese and toppings of choice. Preheat oven to 500 °F. If you have a pizza stone place it in the oven and let it heat. Once oven is at temperature add your pizza either to the hot pizza stone or onto a baking sheet. Baking for 10 – 12 minutes. |

Of course, if you have pizza dough, you need tomato sauce. Below is a quick and simple tomato sauce recipe that makes a great addition to pizza, pasta dishes, and chilies.

## Half Homemade Tomato Sauce

- 1 28-oz. can crushed tomatoes
- 2 tablespoons olive oil
- 3 garlic cloves, minced
- 2 tablespoons of mirepoix (recipe on page 55), or 1 onion, 2 chopped carrots, and 2 chopped celery stalks
- ¼ cup red wine (optional)
- 1 – 2 teaspoons of herbs/spices of choice: oregano, thyme, rosemary, garlic powder
- 2 teaspoons salt
- leftover meat or vegetables*

In a large pot heat olive oil on medium heat. Sauté garlic and mirepoix mixture until tender, roughly 5 minutes. Add red wine and sauté for another 5 minutes. Add crushed tomatoes and simmer for 1 hour without a lid. Add any additional vegetables and/or meat. If a smooth sauce is desired, process it in a blender or use an immersion blender. Add salt and herbs.

*ground beef, chicken, mushrooms, zucchini, and bell peppers make great additions to tomato sauce.

The rest of the recipes are simple and nutritious meal ideas that utilize frequently leftover ingredients.

## Any Leftover Ingredient Frittata

- 3 tablespoons olive oil
- 8 large eggs
- ½ cup milk
- ½ teaspoon salt
- ¼ teaspoon black pepper
- 1 cup leftover ingredients (vegetables, meats, potatoes, cheese, rice, or quinoa)

Preheat oven to 350°F. Heat a 10-inch to 13-inch oven-safe skillet over medium heat. Add olive oil and your leftover ingredients. Sauté until softened. Meanwhile, beat eggs, milk, salt, and pepper in a large bowl. Pour egg mixture into the skillet and cook on stovetop for 5 minutes. Then place the skillet in the oven. Bake for 15-20 minutes or until set.

## Kitchen Sink Soup (Includes Freezing Instructions)

Soup is one of the best meals to make with leftover vegetables. It is also a great way to use vegetables that you no longer want to eat raw. Vegetable soup is a great way to start a meal. The hot broth fills you up and depending on the ingredients you add, you can easily consume several servings of vegetables. You do not need to follow a recipe 100%, which means that most beginner home cooks can make a great tasting soup.

- 2 tablespoons of olive oil
- ½ cup of mirepoix
- 4 – 6 cups of water or broth*
- 1 – 2 cups of any leftover vegetable, leftover starches (rice, pasta, beans), and leftover proteins (meats, poultry, beans). Beans and meats should be cooked already. Rice and pasta can be dry.
- 1 bay leaf
- salt and pepper to taste

* If you are using water, you may want to add more seasoning such as black pepper, salt, garlic powder or dried herbs such as parsley and dill.

Heat a large pot containing olive oil on medium. Add mirepoix and sauté for 4 minutes or until tender. Add the water or broth and then add the leftover ingredients. Then add the bay leaf and cook for about an hour on a low boil. Season with salt and pepper

1. Once cooked, cool the soup completely. If it takes more than 2 hours, place the soup in the refrigerator. (Remember temperature danger zone!)
2. Once cooled, scoop the soup into quart-size freezer bags and seal.
3. Lay the bags of soup flat in the freezer.
4. When you are ready to eat it, simply defrost the soup and re-heat.

## Vegetable/Meat Casserole

- 2 cups cooked rice
- 1 cup cooked quinoa
- 2 cups cheese (cottage cheese, cheddar, mozzarella)
- 2 eggs
- 1 teaspoon black pepper
- 2 cups vegetables/meat of choice
- 1 tablespoon olive oil

Preheat oven to 400°F. In a large bowl mix cheese, eggs and pepper. Mix in the rice and quinoa then add the vegetables/meat. Pour the mixture into a greased baking dish. Cook for 40 minutes.

## Leftover Vegetable or Meat Stock

Stock/broth is very easy to make, and much cheaper than purchasing it at the grocery store. Freeze leftover vegetables, stalks, or pieces that you would otherwise throw away, such as the skin of carrots, in quart size freezer bags. When the bag is full, make your broth.

- 2 tablespoons of olive oil
- 2 medium carrots
- 2 medium onions
- 3 stalks of celery
- 1 – 2 cups of leftover vegetable scraps
- 3 – 4 lbs of mixed bones (beef, pork, chicken)*

In a large pot add about ¼ cup of olive oil. Add a chopped onion. Sauté for 5 minutes. Add the vegetables from your freezer bag and cover with water. Simmer the mixture for 45 minutes. Add salt to taste. Discard the vegetables or compost. See chapter 8 for composting tips. The broth can be frozen in portions in a mason jar or in freezer bags.

* If making beef or chicken stock, roast the bones that you have at 450ºF for 25-30 minutes, or until brown. Add the bones to the pot right after you add the vegetables and bring to a simmer along with the vegetables.

## Smoothies

Smoothies can be made with pretty much any fruit you have on hand. Extremely ripe fruit that you would not normally want to eat by itself, such as bruised bananas or berries that have been squished are great for smoothies. When selecting ingredients for smoothies, try to include a protein to balance the sugar and carbohydrates from the fruit. Adding a protein will make the smoothie more filling and satisfying.

- 1 cup fruit of choice
- 2 cups water, milk, or ice
- 1 cup yogurt (plain preferably)

Protein additions
- ¼ cup peanut butter or nuts
- ½ - 1 cup of Silken tofu
- 1 - 2 tablespoon of flax seeds or chia seeds

Blend until smooth.

## Any Ingredient Tacos

Tacos are an easy meal option. The key ingredients in great-tasting tacos are healthy proteins, lots of vegetables, and a tasty sauce. Any additional toppings or herbs, like cilantro, can easily be added to your tacos. Adding avocado as a topping or using olive oil as a dressing is a great way to include healthy fats in this meal.

- whole wheat tortillas
- cooked beans, ground beef, chicken, or fish
                         OR
- canned fish *
- vegetables of choice (bell peppers, onions, shredded cabbage, spinach)
- sauce of choice for topping: salsa, avocado dressing (see page 70),  yogurt sauce (see page 48)
- cheese of choice (optional)

Cook vegetables if desired. Warm the tortillas in the oven or in the microwave according to package. Assemble tacos by adding each ingredient to the warmed tortilla. Top with sauce of choice.

*Canned fish, such as salmon, goes great with tacos. Simply mixed the canned fish with ¼ cup of plain yogurt and a dash of salt, pepper, and garlic powder.

## Any Ingredient Rice Bowls

Rice bowls are similar to tacos except that rice is used instead of tortillas. The key ingredients in great rice bowls are the same as the key ingredients in tacos: healthy proteins, lots of vegetables, and a tasty sauce. Adding avocado or using olive oil is a great way to include healthy fats in this meal.

- 2 cups cooked rice or quinoa
- 1-2 cups vegetables of choice
- 1 cup of cooked beans, ground beef, chicken, or fish
- sauce of choice: salsa, avocado dressing (see page 70), yogurt sauce (see page 48)

In a bowl add the rice, vegetables and protein of choice. Add sauce on top and enjoy.

## Overnight Oats

Overnight oats are my favorite breakfast. I make it the night before so there is nothing to prepare in the morning. The milk added the night before essentially 'cooks' your oats so they are soft, which means no actual cooking is required.

- ⅓ cup dry rolled oats
- ½ cup of milk of choice
- 2-3 spoonfuls yogurt, preferably plain
- ¼ cup nuts or seeds of choice
- ½-1 cup fruit of choice*
- ½ teaspoon cinnamon
- ½ - 1 teaspoon sweetener, such as honey or maple syrup

Place dry oats in a container. Add the milk, yogurt, fruit, nuts, and cinnamon. Seal container and place it in the refrigerator overnight. Enjoy cold the next morning.

*Any fruit works well. Frozen berries are great to add the night before, because they will defrost by morning. The juice created as they thaw will help sweeten the plain yogurt.


## Any Fruit Yogurt Parfaits

Yogurt parfaits can be a healthy and filling breakfast. Skip purchasing already made fruit and yogurt parfaits, which have a lot of added sugar and cost more than making them at home.

- 1 cup plain yogurt
- ¼ cup nuts
- ½ cup fresh fruit or frozen*
- 1 teaspoon cinnamon
- 1-2 teaspoons maple syrup, honey or jam**

*If you are using frozen fruit, add it to the yogurt the night before you plan to eat it and store it in the refrigerator. Overnight, the fruit will defrost and sweeten the plain yogurt.
**Try to add as little added sugar as possible.

## Sauces/Dressing

Sauces and dressings can make any dish into a delicious meal. Good sauces/dressings are necessary for rice bowls, tacos, and of course salads.

Yogurt Sauce
- 1 cup plain yogurt
- 2 tablespoons fresh herbs of choice
- 1 tablespoon olive oil
- 1 garlic clove, minced
- ¼ teaspoon of both salt and pepper
- ½ lemon, juiced

Mix all ingredients in a food processor or blender.

Vinaigrette-Style Dressings
Try making your own dressing instead of purchasing bottled dressings, which often have a lot of salt and added sugar. The dressings below can be stored at room temperature for about 1 week. Simply mix all ingredients by hand or in a food processor.

Red Wine Vinaigrette Dressing
- ½ cup olive oil
- ⅓ cup red wine vinegar
- 2 teaspoons honey
- dash of salt and pepper

Balsamic Vinaigrette Dressing
- ½ olive oil
- ⅓ balsamic vinegar
- 2 teaspoons fresh mustard
- pinch of salt and pepper

Lemon Vinaigrette dressing
- ½ cup olive oil
- juice and zest of 1 lemon,
- 1 teaspoons garlic powder
- 1 teaspoon oregano

# Ingredient Substitutions

It can be frustrating when a recipe calls for an ingredient you do not have. This can lead to unplanned trips to the grocery store, reaching for unhealthy frozen dinners, or ordering takeout. When you start a recipe and it calls for an ingredient you do not have, try substituting it for a similar ingredient.

TABLE 9. Ingredient Substitutions

| Recipe Calls for | Can be Substituted with |
| --- | --- |
| Breadcrumbs | Cooked Quinoa |
| White Vinegar | Lemon/Lime Juice |
| Tahini | Peanut Butter |
| Brown Sugar | White Sugar |
| Mayonnaise | Plain Yogurt or Cottage Cheese in a Blender |
| Honey | Maple Syrup |
| Fresh Herbs | Dried Herbs |
| Fish Sauce | Worcestershire Sauce or Soy Sauce |
| Oil (in Baking) | Apple Sauce and/or Mashed Bananas |
| Sour Cream | Plain Yogurt |
| Cream/Half-and-Half | Whole Milk |
| Cottage Cheese | Ricotta Cheese or Plain Yogurt |
| Cornstarch (for thickening) | Flour |
| Buttermilk | Milk Plus One Teaspoon of Vinegar/Lemon juice mixed |
| All-Purpose Flour | Whole Wheat Flour (I use whole wheat flour in everything and it always comes out good.) |
| Coconut Milk | Dairy Milk |

# Getting Started with Frozen Produce

If you are not used to cooking with fresh produce, or find yourself frequently wasting fresh vegetables try cooking with frozen produce. Frozen produce often have similar nutritional values to fresh vegetables because they are flash frozen at peak of ripeness.[35]

Frozen produce is a great way to get into the habit of adding vegetables to your daily meals. Frozen vegetables are already precut and do not take much time or effort to prepare. When purchasing frozen produce, be sure to read the ingredients to make sure the produce only contains vegetables and does not contain added sugars, salt, or sauces.

Adding frozen vegetables to mixed dishes like casseroles, frittatas, soups or muffins are a great way to use them. Simply thaw the vegetables by running them under cold water then add them to your dish. Since frozen vegetables are usually blanched, there is no need to cook them beforehand. Once you get used to using frozen produce, you can then transfer to using fresh produce if desired.

Below are storage tips, cooking methods, and some additional recipes for common ingredients.

# Additional Sweet and Savory Recipes

## Vegetables

### Fresh Greens

*How to Store*

Have you ever been excited about making a healthy salad only to find slimy, wilted greens waiting for you in the refrigerator? Loose, leafy greens are one of the harder vegetables to keep fresh. Fresh greens, like bagged salad, can spoil quickly. After some experimenting, talking with others, and doing some research, I have found that the best ways to keep leafy greens fresh is to put the unwashed greens in a container with a paper towel and close the lid. The paper towel will absorb moisture while the container keeps the greens from getting squished and releasing moisture that would make them wilt.

For bunches of greens that include a stem, such as kale, bok choy, swiss chard, or collard greens, I find that placing them in an open plastic bag works best.

| TABLE 10. How to Freeze/Preserve Fresh Greens | | |
|---|---|---|
| Preservation Method | Instructions | Uses |
| Blanch* and Freeze | Cut leafy greens to desired length. Blanch for 1 minute. Freeze individually on a cookie sheet or plate. Place in freezer bag for storage. | Soups/Stews |
| Bake (kale) | Try kale chips ( see recipe below). Store kale chips in a brown paper bag or in an airtight container | Healthy Snacks |
| Cook and Freeze | Try kale pesto, (see recipe below). Cool the pesto and place in a glass container. (Mason jars work great.) | Pizza Spread, Pastas |

*Blanching kills enzymes in the food that would further the ripening process.

| TABLE 11. How to Blanch |
|---|
| 1. Bring 1 gallon of water to a boil |
| 2. Drop vegetables into the water. When possible, use a basket. |
| 3. After boiling for the recommended time (provided in specific produce sections), place the vegetables in an ice bath and let them cool. |
| 4. Freeze as instructed. |

*Quick Nutritious Recipes*

**Kale Pesto**
- ⅓ cup walnuts or pine nuts, toasted
- 3 cups chopped kale
- ½ cup grated parmesan cheese
- ½ cup extra virgin olive oil
- ¼ teaspoon salt

Add kale and salt to a food processor then pulse until chopped. Add the olive oil and parmesan cheese and pulse until combined. Transfer the kale pesto to an airtight container and store in the refrigerator or freezer.

**Kale Chips**
- 1 bunch kale
- 1 teaspoon olive oil
- seasoning of choice

Preheat oven to 300°F. Remove the leaves from the stems. Wash and dry the leaves thoroughly. Drizzle with olive oil and sprinkle with seasoning of choice. Place kale onto a baking sheet. Make sure not to overlap the kale pieces. Bake until crispy, roughly 10-15 minutes.

**Basic Dark Leafy Green Sauté**
- 1 bunch dark, leafy greens
- 1 teaspoon olive oil
- 2 garlic cloves, minced (or 2 teaspoons of garlic powder)

In a skillet or pan, heat oil over medium heat. Add garlic, stir, and cook for 40 seconds. Add greens and cook for another 2 – 5 minutes or until slightly wilted.

| Reminder! |
| --- |
| Do not forget about making pizza, soup, frittata, rice bowls, and tacos. |

# Broccoli and Cauliflower

*How to Store*

Place vegetables in the crisper drawer in the refrigerator. To prolong storage, wrap them in a paper towel and refrigerate them in an open or perforated plastic bag.

| TABLE 12. How to Freeze/Preserve Broccoli and Cauliflower | | |
|---|---|---|
| Preservation Method | Instructions | Uses |
| Blanch and Freeze | Cut broccoli or cauliflower into 1½ inch florets. Blanch for 3 minutes. Freeze individually on a cookie sheet or plate then store in freezer bags. | Soups, Casseroles, Frittatas, or Side dishes |

*Quick Nutritious Recipes*

**Roasted Cauliflower and Broccoli with Quinoa and Tahini sauce**
- 2 small broccoli crowns
- 1 small cauliflower
- 1 cup quinoa cooked according to package

Tahini Sauce
- ½ cup tahini
- ½ cup water
- 2 tablespoons rice vinegar or white distilled vinegar
- 2 tablespoons soy sauce
- 2 garlic cloves
- 1 teaspoon freshly grated ginger or ginger powder

Preheat oven to 400°F. Chop broccoli and cauliflower into bite-size pieces and place on a baking sheet. Drizzle olive oil over the vegetables. Roast for 30 minutes or until soft. In a food processor mix the tahini, water, rice vinegar, soy sauce, garlic cloves, and ginger. If you would like your sauce to be thinner, add more water. Add cooked quinoa and vegetables to a large bowl. Pour tahini sauce over the entire mixture.

**Cauliflower Rice Crumble**

- 1 head cauliflower

Remove any stems or leaves from cauliflower. Cut cauliflower into small pieces. Grate cauliflower with a cheese grater or food processor. Once cauliflower is crumbly and resembles rice, transfer it to a clean towel and squeeze out any moisture. The "rice" can be used raw or can be cooked. To cook, heat a skillet over medium heat and add a tablespoon of butter or olive oil. Add the cauliflower and a dash of salt. Cover the skillet and cook for 5 – 8 minutes or until tender as you would like.

| Reminder! |
| --- |
| Do not forget about making pizza, soups, frittatas, rice bowls, and tacos. |

# Root Vegetables

*How to Store*

Root vegetables can be stored for a long time in a refrigerator or cellar, if you have one. If you purchase root vegetables with tops on them, such as beets and carrots cut the tops off. If you leave the tops on, water will be drawn to the vegetables, which will cause them to shrivel and spoil quicker.

Placing carrots (both regular and baby carrots) and celery in cold water helps to keep them fresh and crisp. Change the water when it starts to look cloudy. If you do not want to deal with the water, place them in an airtight container with a paper towel.

| Table 13. How to Freeze/Preserve Root Vegetables Carrots and Celery | | |
|---|---|---|
| Preservation Method | Instructions | Uses |
| Cook and Freeze (Mirepoix) | Mirepoix is a base that is used for soups, stock, sauces, and stews. To make mirepoix, see the recipe below. Spread mirepoix on a cookie sheet or plate and freeze individually. Store in the freezer until needed. | Soups, Stocks, Sauces, and Stews |

*Quick Nutritious Recipes*

**Mirepoix**
Makes 1 pound
- ½ lb onion, chopped
- ¼ lb cup celery, chopped
- ¼ lb Cut all the ingredients into ¼-inch pieces. Use mirepoix as a base for soups, stocks, sauces, and stews. Mirepoix can be used fresh or frozen for later use.

**Carrot and Date Mini Muffins**
Makes approximately 30 mini muffins (or 15 regular-size muffins)
- 2 cups whole wheat flour
- 2 large carrots, shredded or grated on a cheese grater
- 1 teaspoon baking powder
- 1 egg
- ½ cup shredded coconut

- 1 teaspoon vanilla extract
- 2 teaspoons ground cinnamon
- 7 medjool dates, pitted
- ¼ cup orange juice
- 1 ½ cups apple sauce
- 1 cup water
- 1 cup of walnuts chopped (optional)

Preheat oven to 350ºF. Sift the flour, baking powder, and cinnamon. Set aside. In a food processor, blend pitted dates and ½ cup of applesauce for 1 minute. In a large bowl, mix 1 cup of apple sauce, vanilla extract, carrots, blended dates mixture, and egg. Alternate mixing ½ cup of flour mixture with ¼ cup of water, until all of the flour mixture and water have been combined. If you are adding walnuts fold them into in the batter. Drop spoonfuls of the batter into a greased muffin tin up to the rim. Bake mini muffins for 20 minutes. (Bake regular-size muffins for 25 minutes.) Allow muffins to cool for 5 minutes. Remove them from the pan and allow them to cool on a cooling rack for an additional 10 minutes.

## Beet and Carrot Coleslaw
Makes approximately 4 servings

- 1 lb beets (about 3 medium beets)
- ½ lb carrots (about 3)
- 2 tablespoons of olive oil
- 4 tablespoons of red wine vinegar
- 2 tablespoons of Dijon mustard
- pinch of salt
- 3 tablespoons of fresh parsley chopped (optional)

Peel carrots and beets and grate them on a box grater. A food processor will also work well. In a separate bowl combine the olive oil, red wine vinegar, mustard and salt. Pour dressing over the carrot and beet mixture. Sprinkle parsley if using on top. Store in the refrigerator until cold (about an hour) and then enjoy.

## Beet Hummus
Makes approximately 12 side servings
- 2 small cooked and peeled beets chopped
- 2 (15-oz.) cans chickpeas drained and rinsed
- 1/3 cup tahini
- 2 garlic cloves chopped
- ¼ cup lemon juice
- pinch of salt

Add all ingredients to a food processor and process until smooth. Serve with pita bread, additional vegetables or as a topping for a sandwich

| Reminder! |
| --- |
| Grated carrots and beets would be great in a rice bowl or in tacos. |

# Mushrooms

*How to Store*

If mushrooms were purchased from the store pre-packaged, put them in the refrigerator as is. If you purchased unpackaged mushrooms, place them in a brown paper bag and store them in the refrigerator.

| TABLE 14. How to Freeze/Preserve Mushrooms | | |
|---|---|---|
| Preservation Method | Instructions | Uses |
| Dehydrate* | Preheat an oven or a food dehydrator to 130-140°F. Dry the mushrooms until brittle. Cool the mushrooms completely, then place them in an airtight container. Store them in a cool place for 2 months. | Soups, Pizza, Casseroles or Pasta |
| Cook and Freeze | Cook sliced, quartered, or whole mushrooms in olive oil until tender. Cool and freeze individually on a cookie sheet or a large plate. Store frozen mushrooms in a freezer bag. | Soups, Pizza, Casseroles or Pasta |

*Rehydrate mushrooms by soaking them in boiling water for 30 minutes. They are ready when they have softened all the way through.

**Healthy Mushroom Sauce**
- 1 cup broth of choice
- 1 cup white wine, optional (If you do not have white wine, use an extra cup of broth.)
- 2 tablespoons butter
- 3 8-ounce packages of white button or portobello mushrooms, washed and chopped
- 4 large shallots, minced
- 4 large garlic cloves, minced
- 2 tablespoons dried herbs, such as parsley, oregano, sage, or dill
- 3 tablespoons whole wheat flour
- pinch of salt and fresh ground black pepper

Melt the butter in a large skillet Add the garlic and shallots and sauté for 3 minutes. Add the mushrooms. Sprinkle the flour over the mushrooms and mix until the mushrooms are evenly coated. Add broth and wine to the pot. Bring the mixture to a simmer. Stir frequently until the sauce is thickened, about 15 minutes. Add the herbs and spices. Enjoy this sauce over rice, chicken, beef, fish, or vegetables.

| Reminder! |
|---|
| Do not forget about making pizza, soup, frittata, rice bowls, and tacos. |

# Summary Squash (includes zucchini and yellow squash)

*How to Store*

Place unwashed summer squash and zucchini in a perforated plastic bag or an untied plastic bag in the refrigerator. Place in the crisper drawer.

| Table 15. How to Freeze/Preserve Summer Squash | | |
|---|---|---|
| Preservation Method | Instructions | Uses |
| Blanch and Freeze | Slice zucchini and squash into 1-inch slices. Blanch for 3 minutes. Freeze individually on a cookie sheet or plate. Store in freezer bags. | Cooked Dishes such as casseroles and soups. |

*Quick Nutritious Recipes*

**Zucchini Cakes**
- 1 pound (about 2 medium) zucchini
- 1 teaspoon coarse or kosher salt, plus extra to taste
- 1 large egg, lightly beaten
- 1 teaspoon freshly ground black pepper
- ½ cup all-purpose flour
- ½ teaspoon baking powder
- 2 tablespoons of canola oil (if frying)

Grate the zucchini with a box grater. Place the zucchini in a clean dish towel or cheese cloth and squeeze out as much liquid as you can. Dry zucchini cakes will hold together better. In a large bowl, mix the grated zucchini with the rest of the ingredients. Form mixture into patties. Bake or panfry the patties. If baking, preheat oven to 350°F. Place patties on a baking sheet. Bake for 15 minutes or until golden brown. If panfrying, add canola oil to a skillet. Add zucchini patties to the pan and cook for 7 minutes. Carefully flip the zucchini cakes and cook them for an additional 5 minutes.

## Chocolate Zucchini Muffins

Makes approximately 20 muffins

- 1 cup sugar
- ½ cup applesauce
- 3 large eggs
- 2 teaspoons pure vanilla extract
- 2 ½ cups whole wheat flour
- ½ cup unsweetened cocoa powder
- 1 teaspoon salt
- 1 teaspoon baking soda
- 1 teaspoon ground cinnamon
- 2 cups finely grated zucchini, slightly drained
- 1 cup semisweet chocolate chips

Preheat oven to 350ºF. Grease a muffin pan. Mix the dry ingredients in a large bowl. In a separate bowl, mix the eggs, applesauce, sugar, and vanilla extract. Gradually add the wet ingredients to the dry ingredients. Add the zucchini and mix until well combined. Add the chocolate chips. Scoop the batter into the muffin pan. Bake for approximately 20 minutes. The muffins are done when a knife inserted in the center of the muffin comes out clean.

| Reminder! |
| --- |
| Do not forget about making pizza, soup, frittata, rice bowls, and tacos. |

# Winter squash

*How to Store*

Winter squash does not need to be refrigerated. It can be stored in a cool, dry area of your house for 3 months or longer.

| TABLE 16. How to Freeze/Preserve Winter Squash | | |
|---|---|---|
| Preservation Method | Instructions | Uses |
| Puree and Freeze | To make squash puree, see recipe below. Cool puree then place it in an airtight container or freezer bag | Baked Goods, Pies, and Creamy Soups |

*Quick Nutritious Recipes*

**Winter Squash and Coconut Milk Soup**
- 2 medium types of winter squash (butternut, kabocha, pumpkin, or sweet potatoes), peeled and cut into pieces
- 1 medium onion, chopped
- 1 13-oz. can coconut milk (full fat)
- approximately 2 cups vegetable broth
- 1 tablespoon rosemary
- 1 teaspoon nutmeg
- dash of salt
- 1 teaspoon black pepper
- 2 tablespoons olive oil

Preheat oven to 400°F. Roast butternut squash and/or sweet potatoes until almost fully cooked through (roughly 25 minutes). Remove the squash from the oven. In a large pot, heat olive oil and sauté the onions. Add the squash and sweet potato, coconut milk, and vegetable stock. Cook for twenty minutes, or until the vegetables are soft. Puree the soup with an immersion blender or high-speed blender. Return the puree to the pot and add the seasoning. Cook for an additional 10 minutes on very low heat.

**Butternut Squash Mac and Cheese**
- 1 cup of dry such as rigatoni, penne or elbows
- 1 tablespoon olive oil or butter
- 1 small yellow onion, sliced
- 1 small butternut squash, cubed (4-5 cups)

- 5 cups chicken or vegetable broth
- ¾ cup milk
- 1 teaspoon salt
- ⅔ cup shredded cheese
- salt and pepper to taste

Melt the butter in a saucepan. Add the sliced onions and sauté. Add the broth, milk, and butternut squash and cover. Cook until the butternut squash can be pierced with a fork, approximately 25 minutes. While the butternut squash is cooking, cook pasta according to directions. If you do not mind a chunky cheese sauce, simply mash the squash with a fork. For a smoother sauce, transfer the sauce to a blender. Add the sauce to the cooked pasta and top with cheese, salt, and pepper. Enjoy!

**Basic Squash Puree**

Ingredients
- two winter squash (butternut, pumpkin, acorn, hubbard, kabocha)
- 4 tablespoons of softened butter
- pinch of salt and pepper to taste

Preheat the oven to 350 °F. Cut the squash in half lengthwise and remove any seeds and strings. Seeds can be saved and roasted if desired. Rub the inside of each squash with two tablespoons of butter. Season with salt and pepper. Bake for 30 – 40 minutes or until tender. Remove the squash and scoop out the flesh. Puree until smooth. Place in a freezer bag and store.

| Reminder! |
| --- |
| Do not forget about making pizza, soup, frittata, rice bowls, and tacos. |

# Peppers

*How to store*

Place unwashed peppers in a perforated or open plastic bag in the crisper. Green peppers will last longer than red, yellow, or orange peppers because they are not as ripe.

| TABLE 17. How to Freeze/Preserve Peppers | | |
|---|---|---|
| Preservation Method | Instructions | Uses |
| Slice and Freeze | Wash and slice peppers. Freeze individually on a cookie sheet or plate. Store in freezer bags. | Cooked Dishes such as casseroles and soups. Also tastes great cooked in tomato sauce. |

*Quick Nutritious Recipe*

**Stuffed Peppers**
- 6 medium peppers
- 1 teaspoon olive oil
- 2 garlic cloves, chopped
- ½ onion, chopped into ½-inch pieces
- 2 ½ cups cooked brown rice or quinoa
- ½ teaspoon garlic powder
- ¼ teaspoon salt
- ¼ cup of parmesan cheese or ½ cup of other cheese (optional)

Preheat oven to 350ºF. Cut the tops off the peppers and core their insides. Cook peppers in boiling water for 5 minutes then drain them. In a skillet, heat olive oil then add garlic and onion. Sauté until tender, approximately 4 minutes. Add the rice and spices and cook for another 3 minutes. Spoon the rice mixture into each bell pepper and place peppers onto a baking sheet. Bake for 25 minutes. If using parmesan cheese add on top of the peppers right after you take the peppers out o the oven

| Reminder! |
|---|
| Do not forget about making pizza, soup, frittata, rice bowls, and tacos. |

# Onions

## *How to Store*

Onions keep best when stored in an open bag (not plastic) or in a bowl. You can make a simple onion bag by taking a brown paper bag, and poking holes throughout the bag with a hole puncher or scissors. It is best to keep onions away from other vegetables, especially potatoes. Storing the two together will facilitate spoilage.

| TABLE 18. How to Freeze/Preserve Onions | | |
| --- | --- | --- |
| Preservation Method | Instructions | Uses |
| Freeze | Wash your onions, then slice them into ½-inch thick slices. Place individually on a cookie sheet or a large plate. Once frozen place onions into a freezer bag. | Soups, Sauté for dishes such as casseroles. |
| Cook and Freeze (caramelized onions) | To cook caramelized onions, see the recipe below. Cool completely and store in freezer bags. | Topping for salads, pasta dishes, sandwiches and pizza. |

## *Quick Nutritious Recipes*

### Slow Cooker Caramelized Onions
- 3 – 6 teaspoons of olive oil or butter or a combination of both (roughly one teaspoon for each onion)
- 3 – 6 onions sliced

In a crockpot or slow cooker, add the sliced onions and drizzle the olive oil/butter over. Cook on low for 8 – 10 hours.

To cook without a slow cooker, place onions and olive oil/butter mixture in a pan on medium heat. Stir occasionally so the onions do not burn for 1 hour.

| Reminder! |
| --- |
| Do not forget about making pizza, soup, frittata, rice bowls, and tacos. |

# Potatoes

*How to Store*

Potatoes do not need to be refrigerated. Put potatoes in a paper bag and store them in a cool, dry place. Never store potatoes with onions. If you do not have a cool, dry place in your house, or you live in a humid environment, you can store them in the refrigerator. The potatoes may turn starchy and may taste a bit sweeter when stored in the refrigerator.

| TABLE 19. How to Freeze/Preserve Potatoes | | |
|---|---|---|
| Preservation Method | Instructions | Uses |
| Freeze | Slice, peel and cut potatoes into roughly 2" pieces. Blanch for 4 minutes and then place on a cookie sheet or large plate and freeze individually. Once frozen add to freezer bags. | Hash Browns or French Fries. |

*Quick Nutritious Recipes*

**Healthy Fully-Loaded Baked Potatoes**
- 4 medium sweet potatoes
- 1 cup or 1 can black beans
- 1 cup cooked greens finely chopped (spinach, kale, swiss chard)
- ½ cup plain yogurt
- 1 lime, juice and zest
- ¼ teaspoon salt
- 2 tablespoons mustard
- ½ cup chopped chives
- 1 avocado sliced

Preheat the oven to 400°F. Poke holes in the potatoes with a fork. Cook potatoes for 40-60 minutes or until soft. Meanwhile, make a sauce by mixing plain yogurt, lime juice and zest, salt, and mustard. Cook greens. When potatoes are cooked, slice in half. Top the potatoes with beans, yogurt sauce, avocado, chives and greens. Add additional vegetables, if desired.

**Oven Roasted Potatoes**

Get the crispy taste of a potato without frying!

- 4 large potatoes chopped into 1" pieces
- 1 tablespoons olive oil
- 1 – 2 tablespoons of herbs of choice (garlic powder, oregano, basil, parsley, red pepper flakes)
- ½ teaspoon salt

Preheat oven to 450°F. In a large bowl add ingredients and mix until the potatoes are coated with oil. Spread on a baking sheet so the potatoes are not overlapping. Bake for 20-30 minutes. Halfway through cooking turn the potatoes to cook on both sides. If you want your potatoes extra crispy, broil for 2 minutes.

**Crock-Pot Sweet Potatoes**

This is more of a cooking method than a recipe. Sweet potatoes (not white potatoes) cook wonderfully in the Crock-Pot. Simply wash the potatoes, place them in the Crock-Pot, cover, and cook on low for 6-8 hours. No need to add any liquid.

| Reminder! |
| --- |
| Potatoes with skins contain healthy carbohydrates. Use them in soups and frittatas. They are also a great substitute for rice in rice bowls. |

# Tomatoes

*How to Store*

Whole tomatoes should be stored at room temperature until ripe. Once ripe, place in the refrigerator to avoid spoilage. If you have sliced into a tomato, refrigerate any leftovers in an airtight container.

Tomatoes are very easy to freeze. To freeze tomatoes whole, place them in a freezer bags. You can also freeze pureed tomatoes. Pureed tomatoes can be used just like crushed tomatoes. Just don't eat frozen tomatoes raw. They will be pure mush after defrosted.

| Table 20. How to Freeze/Preserve Tomatoes | | |
|---|---|---|
| Preservation Method | Instructions | Uses |
| Freeze, Whole | Place washed tomatoes into a freezer bag. After you have defrosted your frozen tomatoes, wash off the skin under running water. | Sauces, Soups and Stews |
| Freeze, pureed | Placed washed tomatoes in a food processor. Process until the mixture resembles soup. Transfer the puree to freezer bags and lay flat. | Sauce, Soups and Stews. |

*Quick Nutritious Recipe*

**Tomato Soup**
- 4 cups tomatoes (about 10 tomatoes), chopped
- 1 onion, sliced
- 4 garlic cloves minced
- 2 cups broth
- 2 tablespoons butter or ¼ cup of olive oil
- 2 tablespoons flour
- 1 teaspoon salt
- 2 teaspoons white sugar
- 2 tablespoons basil

In a large stockpot, heat olive oil or butter. Add onions, garlic, and flour. Cook until onions are coated with flour. Add the tomatoes and broth. Bring to a boil then simmer for 30 minutes. Process the soup in a food processor or use an immersion blender. Add spices and sugar.

| Reminder! |
| --- |
| Do not forget about turning extra tomatoes into a quick pizza sauce. |

# Avocados

*How to Store*

Unripe avocados should be stored *outside* the refrigerator. Store ripened avocados *inside* the refrigerator.

| Table 23. How to Freeze/Preserve Avocados | | |
|---|---|---|
| Preservation Method | Instructions | Uses |
| Pureed and Frozen* | Wash the avocado. Scoop out the flesh and mash it with a fork. Mix in ½ teaspoon of lemon juice and a pinch of salt. Place the puree into a freezer bag or a mason jar and place in the freezer. | Toast Topping or Guacamole |
| Sliced and Frozen | Wash, peel and slice the avocados into slices or leave as two halves. Freeze individually on a cookie sheet or large plate. | Same as above |

*Freezing avocados changes their texture.

*Quick Nutritious Recipes*

**Healthy Guacamole**
- 3 ripe avocados
- 1 lime or lemon, juiced
- 1 teaspoon salt
- 2 cloves garlic, minced

Cut avocados in half. Discard the pit, scoop out the flesh and mash. Mix the avocado, lemon juice, salt and garlic. Serve and enjoy.

**Avocado Dressing**
- 1 ripe avocado, cut and flesh scooped out
- 1 cup plain yogurt
- 1 clove garlic, minced
- 1 tablespoon lime juice

- ½ teaspoon black pepper
- ¼ teaspoon salt

Blend all ingredients in a food processor until smooth.

**Avocado and Tofu Chocolate Pudding**
Don't be afraid of the ingredients!
Makes 2 8-oz. servings
- ¼ cup milk of choice
- 8 oz. package of silken tofu
- ½ avocado, cut and flesh scooped out
- ¼ – ½ cup maple syrup (amount depends on how sweet you want your pudding)
- ½ cup unsweetened cocoa powder
- ½ cup chocolate chips
- pinch of salt
- 1 teaspoon vanilla extract

Mix all ingredients in a high-power blender. Serve and enjoy.

# Fruits

## Apples and Pears

*How to Store*

Apples can be stored on the counter. Once ripened, they can be placed in the refrigerator in the low-humidity crisper drawer. If you notice one apple is starting to rot, remove it immediately. One bad apple can cause the others to rot more quickly. If you only want to eat half of an apple, simply rub some lemon juice or water on the flesh and place it in an airtight container. Consume it within one to two days.

Applesauce is extremely easy to make and a tasty way to use apples you do not want to eat raw. Applesauce freezes well and can be used in baked goods or smoothies.

| TABLE 22. How to Freeze/Preserve Apples and Pears | | |
|---|---|---|
| Preservation Method | Instructions | Uses |
| Cook and Freeze | To make applesauce, see the recipe below. Cool the applesauce completely and transfer it to an airtight glass container. (Mason jars work great.) Then transfer to the freezer. | Smoothies, Baked Goods or Yogurt Parfaits |

*Quick Nutritious Recipes*

**Cinnamon Applesauce or Pear butter**
- 3 pounds apples or pears (approximately 6), quartered and cored
- 1 lemon, juiced (approximately 2 tablespoons)
- 1 teaspoon cinnamon
- pinch of salt

Combine apples or pears, lemon juice, cinnamon, and salt in a medium saucepan. Bring the mixture to a boil over medium heat. Cover, and cook, stirring occasionally, until the apples have cooked down into a sauce, 20-25 minutes. Use immediately, or refrigerate in an airtight container for up to 1 week.

## Apple crisp

- 5-7 apples, cut into slices
- ¼ cup butter, cut into small pieces
- ⅓ cup rolled oats
- ⅓cup whole wheat flour
- ½ cup brown sugar or maple syrup
- ½ teaspoon cinnamon
- ¼ teaspoon nutmeg
- ½ cup walnuts
- ½ tablespoon of butter to grease the baking dish

Preheat oven to 375°F. In a medium-size bowl, combine flour, sugar/maple syrup, spices, walnuts, and oats. Add butter and mix until crumbly. Do not be afraid to use your hands. Place chopped apples into an 8-inch greased baking dish. Spoon oat mixture on top. Bake for 35 minutes or until brown. Serve warm.


## Red Wine Vinegar Apple Coleslaw

- 1½ cups shredded cabbage (cut in very thin slices, use a cheese grater or use a mandolin)
- ¾ cups shredded carrots
- 1 large apple, grated (use a cheese grater)
- ½ cup red wine vinegar
- ½ cup olive oil
- ¼ cup lemon juice
- ½ teaspoon salt
- ½ teaspoon black pepper

In a large bowl, combine the cabbage, carrots, and apple. In a separate bowl combine the rest of the ingredients for the dressing. Pour over the cabbage mixture and stir until thoroughly combined.

| Reminder! |
| --- |
| Cubed apples are a great topping for yogurt parfaits. Applesauce tastes great in smoothies, cooked in oatmeal or on top of yogurt. |

# Berries

*How to Store*

Berries are a very sensitive fruit that spoil quickly due to their thin skins. If you buy your berries at the supermarket, keep them in their original container. If you purchased them at a farmers' market and they are in a bag or open container, transfer them to a sealable container lined with a paper towel. Leave the lid slightly open.

| Table 23. How to Freeze/Preserve Berries | | |
|---|---|---|
| Preservation Method | Instructions | Uses |
| Freeze | Wash berries and pat or let them air dry. Freeze individually on a cookie sheet or large plate. Store the frozen berries in a freezer bag. | Smoothies, Topping for Plain Yogurt or Parfaits |
| Cook and Freeze | To make a quick jam, see the recipe below. Cool the jam completely then spoon it into a glass container. (Mason jars work great.) | Topping for Toast, Oatmeal, Pancakes, or Waffles |

*Quick Nutritious Recipes*

**Refrigerator Jam**
Homemade jam is such a great recipe to have in your toolbox. You can use any type of berries to make your jam.
- 2 cups berries, washed
- 1 tablespoon lemon juice
- 1 to 2 tablespoons sugar, such as white sugar, maple syrup, or honey (amount depends on level of sweetness desired)

Add berries to a medium saucepan and cook on medium heat. Add lemon juice and sugar. Once the mixture starts to boil, simmer on low heat. Stir often with a wooden spoon until the jam has thickened. This should take about an hour. Spoon jam into mason jars, cool and store in the refrigerator.

**Frozen Berry Coconut Ice Cream**
- 1 quart frozen berries
- 1 can full-fat coconut milk
- 1 handful of basil
- 1 tablespoon maple syrup

Add all ingredients to a high-power blender and process until smooth. Serve and enjoy

| Reminder! |
| --- |
| Do not forget about making smoothies or fruit parfaits |

# Bananas

## How to Store

Store bananas at room temperature. Do not store in plastic bags. If you have a 'banana tree' hang them for maximum storage.

| TABLE 23. How to Freeze/Preserve Bananas | | |
|---|---|---|
| Preservation Method | Instructions | Uses |
| Slice and Freeze | Peel banana and slice to desired thickness. Freeze individual slices on a cookie sheet or plate. Store in a freezer bag. | Smoothies |
| Bake and Freeze | Banana bread freezes wonderfully. To make banana bread, see the recipe below. Cool the loaf completely then wrap it in plastic wrap or store it in an airtight container. | Defrost and enjoy |

## Quick Nutritious Recipe

Banana Bread
- 2 cups whole wheat flour
- ¾ teaspoon baking soda
- ½ teaspoon salt
- 1 cup sugar
- ¼ cup butter, softened
- 2 large eggs
- 1½ cups mashed ripe banana (about 3 bananas)
- ⅓ cup plain yogurt
- 1 teaspoon vanilla extract
- ½ cup walnuts, chopped

Preheat oven to 350°F. Lightly spoon flour into dry measuring cups; level with a knife. Combine the flour, baking soda, and salt, stir with a whisk. Place sugar and butter in a large bowl and beat with a mixer at medium speed until well blended, about 1 minute. Add the eggs, 1 at a time, beating well after each addition. Add banana, yogurt, and vanilla; beat until blended. Add flour mixture; beat at low speed just until moist. Spoon batter into an 8½ x 4½ loaf pan coated with cooking spray. Bake for 1 hour or until a wooden pick inserted in the center comes out clean. Cool 10 minutes in pan on a wire rack; remove from pan. Cool completely on wire rack.

| Reminder! |
| --- |
| Do not forget about making smoothies or fruit parfaits. |

# Stone Fruits

*How to Store*

Stone fruits, such as peaches and nectarines, are another type of fruit that spoils quickly. Store stone fruits on the counter until they ripen then refrigerate them in a plastic bag unwashed. They will last approximately 2 to 3 days in the refrigerator.

When I have stone fruits that are starting to get too soft, I like to cook them down to a jam (see recipe below). This jam can be stored in a glass container for about one week. It can also be frozen for up to a year.

| TABLE 25. How to Freeze/Preserve Stone Fruits | | |
|---|---|---|
| Preservation Method | Instructions | Uses |
| Cook and Freeze | To make quick jam, see the recipe below. Cool the jam completely then store it in an airtight glass container. (Mason jars work great.) | Smoothies, or Topping for Yogurt, Pancakes, or Sweet Breads. |
| Slice and Freeze | Both peeled and unpeeled fruit can be frozen. Remove stone and slice fruit. Freeze individual slices on a cookie sheet or plate. Store frozen fruit in a freezer bag. | Smoothies |

*Quick Nutritious Recipes*

**Quick Refrigerator Jam**
Homemade jam is such a great recipe to have in your toolbox. It can be used be used on toast, meats, yogurt, oatmeal and smoothies.
- 2 cups stone fruits, sliced and washed. (no need to peel)
- 1 tablespoon lemon juice
- 1-2 tablespoons sugar, such as white sugar, maple syrup, or honey (amount depends on level of sweetness desired)

Add stone fruits to a medium saucepan and cook on medium heat. Add lemon juice and sugar. Once the mixture starts to boil, simmer on low heat. Stir often with a wooden spoon until the jam has thickened, approximately 1 hour. Spoon jam into mason jars, cool and store in the refrigerator.

**Peach or Plum Crisp**
- 4 cups peaches or plums (or both), sliced
- ½ cup whole wheat flour
- ½ cup of cold butter (1 stick), cut into pieces
- 1 teaspoon cinnamon
- ¼ teaspoon salt
- 1 cup rolled oats

Preheat oven to 350°F. In a bowl, mix the flour, oats, sugar, butter, cinnamon and salt with your hands or a pastry cutter until crumbly. Add the peaches/plums to a greased baking dish. Sprinkle the butter mixture over the peaches/plums. Bake for about 30 minutes or until topping is brown.

| Reminder! |
| --- |
| Do not forget about making smoothies or fruit parfaits. |

# Melons

*How to Store*

Melons should be stored at room temperature until they ripen (about 3 days). Melons are ripe when they smell sweet. Ripened melons can be stored in the refrigerator for 1 to 2 days.

When you are ready to cut your melon, make sure to wash it first. Melons may be contaminated with E. coli on their rinds. Inserting a knife into an unwashed melon can spread E. coli to the fruit, which can make you sick. Refrigerate any leftover melon in an airtight container.

| Table 26. How to Freeze/Preserve Melons | | |
|---|---|---|
| Preservation Method | Instructions | Uses |
| Slice and Freeze | Slice melon into bite-size pieces or scoop it out with an ice cream scooper. Freeze individual slices or scoops on a cookie sheet or plate. Store frozen melon in a freezer bag. | Frozen Treats or Smoothies |

*Quick Nutritious Recipe*

**Watermelon and Feta Salad**
- 4-6 cups watermelon
- 1 cup feta cheese
- 1 tablespoon olive oil
- 2 tablespoons lime juice
- ¼ cup chopped fresh mint

Mix all ingredients in a large bowl. Serve cold.

| Reminder! |
|---|
| Do not forget about making smoothies or fruit parfaits. |

# Meats and Poultry

*How to Store*

Raw meats should be stored in its original packaging or in a plastic bag and then placed on the bottom shelf of the refrigerator.

| TABLE 27. How to Freeze/Preserve Meats and Poultry | | |
|---|---|---|
| Preservation Method | Instruction | Uses |
| Freeze, Raw | Tightly wrap raw meat or poultry in plastic wrap then place it in a freezer bag and freeze. Alternatively, keep the meat or poultry in its original package. Store the packaged meat in a freezer bag. | Safely defrost and cook according to recipe/directions |

*Quick Nutritious Recipes*

**Whole Roasted Chicken**
- 1 whole chicken, rinsed and patted dry
- ¾ cups butter, softened
- 3 lemons
- 4 sprigs fresh rosemary or thyme (dried works fine)
- salt and black pepper to taste

Preheat oven to 425°F. Zest two of the lemons. Strip the leaves off of one of the rosemary sprigs and chop them finely. In a bowl, combine softened butter, lemon zest, salt, pepper, and herbs. Rub the chicken with the butter mixture. Pour juice from one lemon over the chicken. Place the other halves of the cut lemons inside the cavity. Roast the chicken for 1 hour and 15 minutes or until the internal temperature is 165 °F. The skin should be a deep golden brown and the juices should be sizzling. Carve and enjoy!

## Beef and Lentil Stew

- 2 tablespoons olive oil
- ½ pound ground beef
- 1 cup lentils
- 1 28-oz. can diced tomatoes
- 1 cup water
- 3 garlic cloves
- 5 carrots, chopped
- 3 celery stalks, chopped
- 1 large onion chopped
- 2 tablespoons of dried or fresh herbs (oregano, parsley, rosemary, thyme)
- salt and pepper to taste

In a large pot, heat olive oil on medium heat. Add the onions, celery, and carrots. Sauté for 5 minutes or until the onions are soft. Add the ground beef and cook for 5 minutes. Add the lentils, diced tomatoes, and water. Cook uncovered for about 20 minutes. Add spices to taste.

| Reminder! |
|---|
| Do not forget about making rice bowls, tacos and pizza. |

# Cheese

*How to Store*

Hard cheeses such as cheddar need to 'breathe.' Tight plastic wrap can cause them to lose their flavor. Wrap hard cheese in parchment paper then storev loosely in a plastic bag on an upper shelf in the refrigerator.

Soft cheese should be stored in an airtight container. Most fresh mozzarella is sold in airtight containers filled with water. If you purchase fresh mozzarella in packaging that does not contain water, add some water to the cheese to keep it fresh.

*How to Freeze/Preserve*

Fresh cheeses do not freeze well, and considering how long they last if stored properly it is not needed. Cooked dishes containing cheese can be frozen successfully.

*Quick Nutritious Recipe*

**Veggie-Filled Grilled Cheese**
- 4 slices whole wheat bread
- 4-6 ounces cheese of choice
- 1 tablespoon room-temperature butter
- ½ cup cooked spinach, onions, mushrooms or other vegetables of choice

Heat a cast iron skillet or other nonstick skillet on medium heat. Assemble your sandwich with the cheese and vegetables. Butter each side of the sandwich and place it on the heated skillet. Cook until golden brown and cheese has melted about 3 – 4 minutes. Flip the sandwich and cook for about 3 minutes on the other side. Cut each sandwich in half and enjoy.

Also see butternut squash mac n cheese on page 62

# Grains

*How to store*

Since whole grains contain both the germ and healthy oils, they will spoil faster than refined grains such as white flour. Store whole grains, such as rice, wheat berries, quinoa and flour in an airtight container in a cool, dry place for up to 6 months.

Rancid flours smell like paint. Flour can also be stored in the refrigerator; however, this is generally not necessary since properly stored flours can last for a long time in a cool, dry place, like a pantry.

| TABLE 28. How to Freeze/Preserve Grains | | |
|---|---|---|
| Preservation Method | Instructions | Uses |
| Freeze | Place flour in an airtight container and store it in the freezer. | Flour does not need to be thawed and can be used as you would normally |

*Quick Nutritious Recipes*

**Croutons**
- 6 slices bread, chopped
- ¼ cup olive oil
- ½ teaspoon garlic powder
- 4 teaspoons oregano or other dried herb of choice

Preheat oven to 375ºF. In a large bowl, add the bread, olive oil, and spices. Mix until the pieces of bread are completely coated. Spread the seasoned bread on a baking sheet. Bake for approximately 10 minutes or until golden brown. Store in an airtight container for up to 2 days at room temperature or freezer for several weeks. Enjoy!

**French Toast**
- 4-6 slices of bread
- 6 eggs
- 1 teaspoon nutmeg
- 1 teaspoon cinnamon
- ½ teaspoon allspice
- ½ teaspoon ground cloves
- 2 tablespoons butter, divided

In a large bowl, beat the eggs and spices. Heat a nonstick skillet on medium heat and grease with butter. Dip a slice of bread into the egg mixture. Place the bread onto the skillet and cook on each side for 3-4 minutes. If you have extra egg mixture add on top of the bread and cook.

## Whole Wheat Pancakes
- 1¼ cup whole wheat flour
- 1 cup buttermilk
- 1 egg
- ¼ teaspoon baking soda
- ½ teaspoon baking powder
- ¼ teaspoon salt
- ¼ cup of sugar*

In a large bowl, mix the dry ingredients. In a separate bowl, mix the wet ingredients. Add the wet ingredients to the dry ingredients and mix until combined. If the batter seems too thick, add water or milk by the teaspoon until you reach the desired consistency. Add ½ cup of the batter to a greased skilled. Cook the pancakes until bubbles form in the batter and the edges are slightly brown, about 3 to 6 minutes. Carefully flip the pancakes with a spatula. Cook for an additional 3-5 minutes or until both sides are golden brown. My favorite pancake topping is plain yogurt mixed with a little bit of maple syrup and fruit. The yogurt provides healthy protein while the maple syrup adds a touch of sweetness.

*You do not need to add sugar to the batter if you plan to top your pancakes with maple syrup.

Pancake Variations
Try adding ½ cup of the following:
- butternut squash or sweet potato puree
- applesauce or grated apples/pears
- banana puree

Note: Adding any of the ingredients listed above will change your batter's consistency and may affect cooking times.

# Chapter 8: For Further Reading

## Environmental Impact of Food Waste

The United States spends roughly one billion dollars per year to dispose of food waste. Food leftovers are the largest portion of our waste stream according to the Environmental Protection Agency. This waste includes unconsumed food and food preparation scraps such as vegetable peels.[36]

Food waste has a significant impact on the environment. Growing food requires a lot of inputs, such as water, energy, and fertilizer/animal feed. In America, bringing food to our plates uses 10% of our total energy budget, 50% of land, and 80% of freshwater per year.[37] In fact, agriculture is responsible for one-third of climate change.[38] To make matters worse, 40% of food that is grown is wasted. When we waste food, we are also wasting the inputs used to grow our food [37].

Food is wasted at all stages of the food chain from harvesting in the fields to consumer waste. Fifty-four percent of the world's food waste occurs during the product, post-harvest-handling, and storage phases. The other forty-six percent of food waste occurs at the processing, distribution, and consumption level.[39]

Sending food to the landfill increases the release of methane gas, a potent greenhouse gas, into the environment. Greenhouse gases increase the temperature in the atmosphere and make the oceans more acidic. Acidic oceans cause the death of aquaculture (farming of fish, crustaceans, molluscs and aquatic plants), which reduces the diversity of commonly-consumed fish species. Today more than 1 billion people worldwide rely on aquaculture as a primary source of food.[40]

Produced-but-uneaten food occupies almost 1.4 billion hectares of land in the word. This represents 30% of the world's agricultural land area, the land cleared for growing food. This wasted land is about the size of India and Canada combined.[41] Cutting down arable land increases the amount of carbon dioxide in the atmosphere, which leads to climate change. In addition, when we cut down land in order to raise livestock, we are decreasing habitats of many animals leading to species loss.

Certain foods require more inputs than other foods. Animal proteins, such as meat, poultry, and dairy, require more inputs than vegetables. In the United States 47% of soy and 60% of corn are used for livestock consumption. This soy and corn take up 33% of arable land. Therefore, when we waste animal products we are not only wasting the animal, but also the feed, inputs for feed, and the land used to raise the animal.

The increase in droughts across the globe has made wasting water a significant issue. Since 70% of the world's freshwater is used for agriculture, the food we eat has a large impact on how much water is used or wasted. Animal proteins require the largest amount of water to produce. Consult the chart below to see the water footprint of certain foods.

| Table 29. Data from Waterfootprint.org | |
|---|---|
| Food Item | Gallons of Water needed to produce one pound of food |
| Beef | 2500 – 5000 |
| Chicken | 815 |
| Eggs | 573 |
| Cheese | 896 |
| Pork | 1630 |
| Tofu | 244 |
| Rice | 403 |
| Wheat Bread | 154 |
| Potatoes | 30 |
| Apples | 83 |
| Oranges | 55 |
| Groundnuts | 383 |
| Chocolate | 2847 |

Every time we throw food away, we also throw away the precious water used to create the food. At the retail and consumer level, fruits and vegetables make up 32% of total food waste. Though not as high as animal proteins, vegetarian proteins and plant-based foods require heavy inputs as well. These foods many not need to be fed grain, but they still need water and fertilizer to grow.

Reducing food waste at the consumer level can significantly improve the environment. One way to reduce food waste, and lower your water and carbon footprints, is to send less food to the landfill.

# Introduction to Composting

Reducing food waste is the best choice for the environment, but the next best thing to do with wasted food is to compost. Composting is a process of recycling decomposed organic materials into nutrient-rich soil known as compost. When added to the soil in your garden, compost help plants grow by adding nutrients back into the soil rather than sending them to the landfill .[42]

Food scraps and yard waste are easy-to-compost items. There is no set *recipe* for creating a compost, but it is important to create a balance between green materials (nitrogen) and brown materials (carbon). The recommended ratio of brown materials to green materials is three to one. The following table provides a list of green and brown materials.

| Table 30. Green and Brown Materials for Composting<br>Data from Bonnie Plants |
| --- |
| Green Materials<br><ul><li>Vegetable Scraps</li><li>Fruit Peels (Limit Citrus)</li><li>Coffee Grounds</li><li>Tea Bags/Grounds</li><li>Houseplants</li><li>Weeds (That Have Not Gone to Seed)</li><li>Plant Pruning</li><li>Fresh Grass</li><li>Hair</li><li>Egg Shells</li></ul> |
| Brown Materials<br><ul><li>Dried Leaves</li><li>Newspaper</li><li>Dried Grass</li><li>Shredded Paper</li><li>Coffee Filters</li><li>Pine Needles</li><li>Pizza Boxes</li><li>Paper Bags</li><li>Cardboard Egg Cartons</li><li>Straw</li></ul> |
| Do NOT Compost at Home<br><ul><li>Pet Feces – can transmit diseases</li><li>Meat and Seafood – attracts rodents and other animals</li><li>Whole Raw Eggs – attracts rodents and other animals</li><li>Dairy Products – attracts rodents and other animals</li></ul> |

There are many ways to compost at home. The equipment needed for each style of composting varies. Composting does not require a lot of space. You can even compost inside an apartment. If you manage your compost bin well, it should not attract pests or create unpleasant odors.

Keeping your compost contained in a structure works best. There are many different containers and materials you can use to create a structure for composting, but you must have airflow. You can create airflow by drilling holes in a container or using chicken wire or hardware cloth around your bin.

Turning your compost will help facilitate the process of decomposition. Turning your compost exposes it to air, which will keep your compost pile aerobic. This encourages microbes to decompose the materials. It is recommended that you turn your compost weekly with a pitchfork, but if you miss a week or two your compost pile will be okay.[43]

Keeping your compost pile moist is also important. You can maintain proper moisture by monitoring the amount of rain in your area and watering your compost during dry spells. If your compost pile starts to get too moist, simply add more brown material to absorb the excess moisture.

Check out the following resources to learn more about composting at home:
- Earth Easy: http://eartheasy.com/grow_compost.html
- Environmental Protection Agency: http://www.epa.gov/recycle/composting-home
- How to Build a Compost Bin: http://extension.missouri.edu/p/G6957

# Conclusion

My goal throughout this guidebook has been to make cooking and healthy eating a simple task for you and your family. Healthy eating should not be a stressful activity that requires all of your time, energy, and money. If you use the information in this guidebook, cooking at home and eating healthy will actually save you time and money. All that is required is a basic understanding of nutrition, food safety and a commitment to meal planning.

Most people want to lead healthy lives. I hope I have helped you realize how easy it is to achieve this goal. Every small change you make to your diet will improve your health. Cooking at home and using your ingredients carefully will save both food and money, which is good for your health and your wallet. This guidebook contains a lot of information. Revisit chapters and topics as you make the changes that will improve your health.

Contact Information

Amanda Terillo
Amanda@nutritiousliferds.com
434-872-3285

# Index

# References

Figure References

"Aerobic Composting: Materials and Setup." *AS Recycling.* Accessed January 30, 2016. https://recycling.as.ucsb.edu/composting/home-composting-guide/aerobic-composting-at-home/aerobic-composting-materials-and-setup/.

"Capri Sun Juice Drink". Capri Sun. Accessed January 11, 2016. http://parents.caprisun.com/juice-drinks

"Healthy Eating Plate & Healthy Eating Pyramid." The Nutrition Source. Accessed May 09, 2016. http://www.hsph.harvard.edu/nutritionsource/healthy-eating-plate/.

"Kellogg's Froot Loops Cereal". Kelloggs.  Accessed January 11, 2016. http://www.kelloggs.com/en_US/kellogg-s-froot-loops-cereal-product.html

"Organic Multigrain Pretzel Rings". Utz. Accessed January 11, 2016. http://www.getutz.com/get-snacks/pretzels/organic-pretzels.html

"Mango". Outshine. Accessed January 11, 2016. http://www.outshinesnacks.com/products/bars/mango.aspx

"Snacks". Frito Lay. Accessed January 11, 2016. http://www.fritolay.com/snacks/product-page/simply/cheetos-puffs-simply-white-cheddar-cheese-flavored-snacks


Table References

"How to Create a Compost Pile." *Bonnieplants.com.* Accessed January 30, 2016. https://bonnieplants.com/library/composting-101-how-to-create-a-compost-pile/.

U.S. Department of Health and Human Services and U.S. Department of Agriculture. 2015 – 2020 Dietary Guidelines for Americans. 8th Edition. December 2015. Available at http://health.gov/dietaryguidelines/2015/guidelines/.

Hoeskstra, Arjen. "The Water Footprint of Food." *Water Foot Print.* http://www.waterfootprint.org/Reports/Hoekstra-2008-WaterfootprintFood.pdf. 2008.

# Notes

1. "Leading Causes of Death," *Center for Disease Control and Prevention*, last modified

2. Steve Economides and Annette Economides, *America's Cheapest Family Gets you Right on the Money* (New York: Three Rivers Press, 2007), 6.

3. Garza, Ding, Owensby, and Zizza, "Impulsivity and Fast-Food Consumption: A Cross Sectional Study among Working Adults," *Journal of the Academy of Nutrition and Dietetics* volume, no 1 (2016): 61 - 68, http://dx.doi.org/10.1016/j.jand.2015.05.003.

4. Susan Morrow, "Study Suggests Home Cooking for a Healthier Diet," *Gazette*, last modified January 2015, http://hub.jhu.edu/gazette/2015/january-february/currents-home-cooking-is-healthier.

5. Urban, Weber, Heyman, Schichti, Verstraete, Lowery, Das, Schleicher, Rogers, Economos, Masters, and Roberts, "Energy Contents of Frequently Ordered Restaurant Meals and Comparison with Human Energy Requirements and US Department of Agriculture Database Information: A Multisite Randomized Study," *Journal of the Academy of Nutrition and Dietetics 116, no. 4 (2916): 590 - 598,,* http://dx.doi.org/10.1016/j.jand.2015.11.009.

6. Aol.com Editors, "Do Fast Food Retailers Really Offer Value Meals?," *aol.com*, last modified May 13, 2013, http://www.dailyfinance.com/2013/05/13/did-you-know-fast-food-isnt-cheaper-savings-experiment/.

7. "Safe Food Handling: What You Need to Know," *U.S. Food and Drug Administration*, last updated September 2, 2015, http://www.fda.gov/Food/ResourcesForYou/Consumers/ucm255180.htm.

8. "Refrigeration and Food Safety," *United States Department of Agriculture Food Safety and Inspection Service*, last modified March 23. 2015, http://www.fsis.usda.gov/wps/portal/fsis/topics/food-safety-education/get-answers/food-safety-fact-sheets/safe-food-handling/refrigeration-and-food-safety/ct_index.

9. "Check your Steps," *Foodsafety.gov*, accessed January 2, 2016, http://www.foodsafety.gov/keep/basics/index.html.

10. "Be Smart. Keep Foods Apart. Don't Cross-Contaminate.," *United States Department of Agriculture: Food Safety and Inspection Service*, last modified July 2,

2013, http://www.fsis.usda.gov/wps/portal/fsis/topics/food-safety-education/get-answers/food-safety-fact-sheets/safe-food-handling/be-smart-keep-foods-apart/ct_index.

11. "Leftovers and Food Safety," *United States Department of Agriculture: Food Safety and Inspection Service*, last modified June 15, 2013, http://www.fsis.usda.gov/wps/portal/fsis/topics/food-safety-education/get-answers/food-safety-fact-sheets/safe-food-handling/leftovers-and-food-safety/ct_index.

12. "Food Product Dating," *United States Department of Agriculture: Food Safety and Inspection Service*, last modified March 24, 2015, http://www.fsis.usda.gov/wps/portal/fsis/topics/food-safety-education/get-answers/food-safety-fact-sheets/food-labeling/food-product-dating/food-product-dating.

13. "How are Food Expiration Dates Determined?," *A Dash of Science*, accessed December 20, 2013, http://adashofscience.com/2013/09/09/food-expiration-dates-determined/.

14. "Forgotten in the Fridge," *Institute of Agriculture and Natural Resources,* accessed December 13, 2015, http://food.unl.edu/forgotten-fridge#handling.

15. Peter Walsh, "Study Says a Cluttered House Can Contribute to Obesity," *WRIC.com*, accessed April 30, 2015, http://wric.com/2015/04/30/study-says-a-cluttered-house-can-contribute-to-obesity/.

16. Tara Parker-Pope, "Putting Your Kitchen on a Diet" *The New York Times Well Blog* (blog), last modified March 3, 2008, http://well.blogs.nytimes.com/2008/03/03/putting-your-kitchen-on-a-diet/?_r=1.

17. "Supermarket Facts," *FMI*, accessed December, 15, 2015, http://www.fmi.org/research-resources/supermarket-facts.

18. "What Is the Meaning of Natural on the Label of Food?," *U.S. Food and Drug Administration*, accessed December 14, 2015, http://www.fda.gov/aboutfda/transparency/basics/ucm214868.htm.

19. Amanda Woerner, "What are Natural Flavors, Really?" CNN.com, last modified January 14, 2015, http://www.cnn.com/2015/01/14/health/feat-natural-flavors-explained/.

20. "Whole Grains 101," *Whole Grain Council*, accessed March 7, 2016, http://wholegrainscouncil.org/whole-grains-101.

21. "Guidance for Industry: A Food Labeling Guide (9. Appendix A: Definition of Nutrient Content Claims," *U.S. Food and Drug Administration*, last modified August 20, 2015, http://www.fda.gov/Food/GuidanceRegulation/GuidanceDocumentsRegulatoryInformation/LabelingNutrition/ucm064911.htm.

22. "Guidance for Industry: A Food Labeling Guide (9. Appendix A: Definition of Nutrient Content Claims)," *U.S. Food and Drug Administration*, last modified August 20, 2015, http://www.fda.gov/Food/GuidanceRegulation/GuidanceDocumentsRegulatoryInformation/LabelingNutrition/ucm064911.htm.

23. "Added Sugars," *American Heart Association*, accessed December 14, 2015, http://www.heart.org/HEARTORG/GettingHealthy/NutritionCenter/HealthyEating/Added-Sugars_UCM_305858_Article.jsp#.VnF3J4TzKf4.

24. "Soft Drinks and Disease," *Harvard School of Public Health*, accessed December 14, 2015, http://www.hsph.harvard.edu/nutritionsource/healthy-drinks/soft-drinks-and-disease/#ref46.

25. "The Secrets Behind Your Grocery Store's Layout," *Real Simple*, accessed January 2, 2016, http://www.realsimple.com/food-recipes/shopping-storing/more-shopping-storing/grocery-store-layout/supermarket-layout.

26. Rebecca Rupp, "Surviving the Sneaky Psychology of Supermarkets," *National Geographic: The Plate*, last modified June 15, 2015, http://theplate.nationalgeographic.com/2015/06/15/surviving-the-sneaky-psychology-of-supermarkets/.

27. Lindsay Haskell, "How Grocery Stores Trick Us Into Buying Unhealthy Foods," *Attn:,* last modified November 16, 2014, http://www.attn.com/stories/276/how-grocery-stores-trick-us-buying-unhealthy-foods.

28. Jamie Logie, "Supermarket Psychology: How Grocery Stores Take Steps That Lead You To Spend More," *Regained Wellness,* last modified May 21, 2014, http://www.regainedwellness.com/supermarket-psychology/.

29. Jason Cabler, "Thirteen Ways Supermarkets Trick You Into Spending More Money," *Celebrating Financial Freedom*, accessed February 12 2015, http://www.cfinancialfreedom.com/supermarkets-trick-spending-money/.

30. Charlene Dy, "Is the Grocery Store Ripping You Off?," *CNN.com*, last modified July 9, 2008, http://www.cnn.com/2008/LIVING/personal/07/09/food.bill/index.html?iref=newssearch.

31. Jahns, Scheett, Johnson, Krebs-Smith, Payne, Whigham, Hoverson, and Kranz, "Diet Quality of Items Advertised in Supermarket Sales Circulars Compared to Diets of the US Population, as Assessed by the Healthy Eating Index-2010," Journal of the Academy of Nutrition and Dietetics 116, no. 1 (2015): 115-122, doi: 10.1016/j.jand.2015.09.016. Epub 2015 Oct 23.

32. "USDA and EPA Join with Private Sector, Charitable Organizations to Set Nation's First Food Waste Reduction Goals," United States Department of Agriculture News Release, September 16, 2015, http://www.usda.gov/wps/portal/usda/usdamediafb?contentid=2015/09/0257.xml&printable=true&contentidonly=true, accessed March 16, 2016.

33. Denise Webb, "High Protein Snacking," *Todays Dietitian* 17, no. 6 (2015): 22, http://www.todaysdietitian.com/newarchives/060415p22.shtml.

34. Rhonda Sebastian, Cecilia Wilkinson Enns, and Joseph Goldman, "Snacking Patterns of U.S. Adults: What We Eat in America, NHANES 2007 – 2008," *Food Surveys Research Group*, last modified June, 2011, http://www.ars.usda.gov/SP2UserFiles/Place/80400530/pdf/DBrief/4_adult_snacking_0708.pdf.

35. Joy Rickman, Diane Barrett, and Christine Bruhn, "Nutritional Comparison of Fresh, Frozen and Canned Fruits and Vegetables. Part 1. Vitamins C and B and Phenolic Compounds," *Journal of the Science of Food and Agriculture* 87, (2007): 930 – 944, http://ucce.ucdavis.edu/files/datastore/234-779.pdf.

36. "Food Waste in America," *Society of St. Andrew*, accessed January 30, 2016, http://endhunger.org/food-waste/.

37. Dana Gunders, "Wasted: How America is Losing Up to 40 Percent of Its Food from Farm to Fork to Landfill," *National Resources Defense Council*, last modified August, 2012, http://www.nrdc.org/food/files/wasted-food-IP.pdf.

38. "Agriculture," *Climate Institute*, accessed January 30, 2016, http://www.climate.org/topics/agriculture.html.

39. "Food Wastage Footprints," *FAO*, accessed March 7, 2016, http://www.fao.org/fileadmin/templates/nr/sustainability_pathways/docs/Factsheet_FOOD-WASTAGE.pdf.

40. "What is Ocean Acidification?," *National Oceanic and Atmospheric Administration*, accessed January 30, 2016, http://www.pmel.noaa.gov/co2/story/What+is+Ocean+Acidification%3F.

41. "Food Wastage Footprints," *FAO*, accessed March 7, 2016, http://www.fao.org/fileadmin/templates/nr/sustainability_pathways/docs/Factsheet_FOOD-WASTAGE.pdf.

42. "Composting at Home," *United States Environmental Protection Agency*, last updated April 8, 2016, https://www.epa.gov/recycle/composting-home.

43. "Backyard Composting," *Eco-Cycle*, accessed January 30, 2016, http://www.ecocycle.org/backyard-composting.

www.ingramcontent.com/pod-product-compliance
Lightning Source LLC
Chambersburg PA
CBHW081226280526
45787CB00006B/2539